W9-CWV-975

THE ADMIRABLE SECRETS
OF PHYSICK AND CHYRURGERY

The Admirable Secrets
of Physick and Chyrurgery

Thomas Palmer

EDITED BY THOMAS ROGERS FORBES

YALE UNIVERSITY PRESS
NEW HAVEN AND LONDON

Designed by Sally Harris
and set in Caslon 540 type by Eastern Typesetting Company.
Printed in the United States of America by
BookCrafters, Inc., Chelsea, Michigan.

Library of Congress Cataloging in Publication Data

Palmer, Thomas, 1666?–1743.
The admirable secrets of physick and chyrurgery.

Bibliography: p.
Includes index.
1. Medicine—15th–18th centuries.   2. Medicine—Philosophy—Early works to
1800.   3. Materia medica, Vegetable—Early works to 1800.   I. Forbes, Thomas
Rogers, 1911–   .   II. Title.
R128.7.P15 1984   610'.9744   84–40200
ISBN 0–300–03209–9

The paper in this book meets the guidelines for
permanence and durability of the Committee on
Production Guidelines for Book Longevity
of the Council on Library Resources.

10   9   8   7   6   5   4   3   2   1

For Liz and Tom

Contents

Acknowledgments

MY FIRST KNOWLEDGE of *Admirable Secrets* came through chance encounter and the kindness of Regina Woody. Her husband, a physician, had worked at length on a copy of the 1696 notebook but had died before completing his studies. His wife urged me to prepare Palmer's manuscript for publication. I have done so without reference to Dr. Woody's work and in fact have not seen his transcription, notes, or other writings except for one letter. Any errors are my own. Mrs. Woody generously responded to my inquiries, gave full approval to my plan to transcribe, edit, annotate, and seek publication of the manuscript, and encouraged my labors.

Dr. William Ober of the New York Academy of Medicine likewise supported the project. Richard J. Wolfe of the Countway Library of Harvard University supplied a photocopy of *Admirable Secrets* and gave permission for its publication. To Dr. Carola Greengard, formerly of Yale University, and Professors Howard Needler and Edward Zlotkowski of Wesleyan University, I am much indebted for correcting my translation of the Latin lines on the title page of Palmer's manuscript and for identifying their sources. Edward Tripp, kindest of editors, gave advice and encouragement. Finally, my thanks are due to Cinda D'Addio and June Connolly, who patiently typed and retyped a difficult manuscript.

T. R. F.

New Haven
October 1983

Note

The reader is warned that the uses and actions of the substances and mixtures mentioned in this book may or may not be as alleged by Thomas Palmer or other authorities cited. Indeed, some of the drugs may be harmful. Interested persons should consult a modern textbook of pharmacology or other appropriate source of information.

Introduction

IN THE YEAR 1696 a young man trudges from one small farm to another—he cannot afford to keep a horse—thinking about the sick woman he has just examined and wondering what afflicts the child, suddenly very ill, who waits for him at the next homestead. Is the woman's fever catching? What has produced her hot humor? Did he bleed her sufficiently? He spies the long green leaves and white flowers of a patch of wild garlic in a damp hollow along the path. Pulling up some of the plants, he stuffs their bulbous roots in his deep pocket. A paragraph in Culpeper comes into his mind: "Garlick . . . hot and dry . . . an enemy to all poysons . . . . It provokes Urin and expels wind." The traveler will add the medicinal plant to his store when he finally gets home, for it is up to him to collect the simples—single parts of plants or other objects that can be prescribed by themselves as remedies.

The weary figure is Thomas Palmer. He is also a preacher—a divine, as such were called—but not a very good one. As a medical man he does much better. Probably trained as an apprentice to a doctor, he continues his education by reading such professional volumes as he can borrow and by constantly pondering the problems of the sick men, women, and children he visits. Diagnosis, prognosis, treatment—all are up to him. In his pocket is a notebook in which he jots down the medical miscellany that overflows his memory, especially the almost innumerable remedies. No one could remember it all. He has been permitted to make extensive notes from a manuscript by the eminent Dr. Samuel Fuller, and to these notes young Palmer adds the admonitions he has found in print, as well as his own ideas and observations. All is in the precious notebook which he keeps constantly at hand.

Soon we shall look at Thomas Palmer's vade mecum, *The Admirable Secrets of Physick and Chyrurgery*. It is a remarkable little book, partly because, completed in 1696, it appears to be the earliest such

1

document to have been written in New England. Palmer's record, assembled for his own use, of what he felt to be most important in physic and surgery preserves for us the epitome of the practice of a busy colonial practitioner at the end of the seventeenth century. We are dependent on sources like Palmer's little book; as J. Worth Estes has observed, "Most of what we know about the practice of medicine in eighteenth-century America has come from what colonial doctors said they did or what they recommended that others do."[1]

Before we open the pages of *Admirable Secrets*, however, it may be helpful to look briefly at the background and nature of colonial medicine.

Sixteenth-Century Medicine

Contemporary additions to medical learning were infrequent and exceptional. Most of what medical men knew was of ancient origin, having been propounded by Hippocrates and Aristotle, supplemented by Galen, and preserved without very much change through the Middle Ages. The concept of specific diseases had not yet really appeared. The patient had a fever or a flux, an apostume or an atrophy. Most such afflictions were seen as secondary to an imbalance in the body's humors, a belief that went back to Galen. The idea was that all things were composed of four elements: air, fire, earth, and water. The elements in turn were responsible for the basic qualities of dryness, heat, cold, and wetness. Within the human body the elements were represented by corresponding humors—yellow bile (air), blood (fire), black bile (earth), and phlegm (water). Of course there were many kinds of people, but this was because the humors were present in different proportions, with one more or less preponderant. An individual might be choleric (yellow bile predominating), sanguine (blood), melancholy (black bile), or phlegmatic (water). Thus has tradition left its stamp on our language.

Sickness resulted when an individual's usual balance of humors

1. J. Worth Estes, "Therapeutic Practice in Colonial New England," in *Medicine in Colonial Massachusetts 1620–1820*, ed. Philip Cash et al., p. 289.

was altered. It followed that it was up to his medical man to find out which humors were wanting or in excess, and to what degree. The hue of the patient's skin, eyes, and urine could be clues, for each humor had its distinctive color. Medicines likewise were classified as hot or cold, moist or dry, and according to the degree to which these qualities were present. Thus, for example, Culpeper spoke of the dwarf elder, *Sambucus*, as "Hot and dry in the third degree," while mallows, *Malva*, were "cold and moist in the first degree."[2] So the doctor selected remedies calculated to restore the patient's humoral balance.

But the humors were not all. In the body there moved three kinds of spirits. Natural spirits were produced in the liver, then transported to the heart and mixed with air to become vital spirits. The latter, carried to the head via the arteries, became animal spirits. Illness would ensue if the accustomed proportions of the spirits were disturbed. Once more it was up to the medical man to restore the proper balance.

As if all this were not enough, he had also to reckon with outside influences—miasma, or noxious vapor, arising at night from the rotting vegetation in a swamp; contagion; and particularly the powerful effects of the planets in their conjunctions. Astrology was of great importance on the medical scene. Aristotle had taught that man the microcosm was under the sway of the macrocosm, ruled by the great heavenly bodies that also controlled the seasons, the tides, growth, and life itself. Over the centuries man had decided that a particular planet regulated each humor and also each part, each organ, of his body; these influences were summarized in useful anatomical diagrams of Zodiacal Man. Equally important, as we shall see, could be the conjunctions—the proximities—of the heavenly bodies. In some conjunctions it was beneficial to purge or bleed; in others, dangerous. Even the simples that became ingredients of the innumerable receipts or prescriptions were best picked with due attention to which planet was then in the ascendancy. Fevers and other afflictions were themselves classified according to the heavenly bodies

2. Nicholas Culpeper, *Pharmacopoeia Londinensis*, pp. 5, 31.

that controlled them. Thus an ailment could be "martial" or "saturnine" or "jovial".[3]

The somnolence of sixteenth-century medical thought was noisily interrupted by an extraordinary Swiss physician, Theophrastus Bombastus von Hohenheim (1493–1541), better known as Paracelsus, and his followers. Paracelsus was irascible, unpolished, dissipated, inconsistent, but also brilliant, original, and iconoclastic, and his ideas seem to have been as disturbing as his personality. He opposed bloodletting and favored a "chemiatric" system for therapy. He saw the human frame as a chemical compound of salt, sulphur, and mercury. When the balance between these was disturbed, illness followed.

The idea of sulphur and mercury as two elemental substances had been propounded much earlier by the alchemists. Debus states that Paracelsus's contribution "was to add salt as the third principle and extend the theory so that it might be used for all things rather than the metals alone." The three elements represented spiritual entities. Mercury embodied volatility, unchangeability in fire, and spirit and water. Sulphur represented inflammability, vaporescence, mutability in fire, and soul and air. Salt connoted noninflammability, unalterability, the residue in ashes, and body and earth.[4]

In practical terms, Paracelsus said, illness might be treated "chemiatrically" by the administration of compounds of iron, lead, mercury, sulphur, copper, and arsenic, together with alcoholic extracts, or tinctures, and mineral baths.[5] He also taught the therapeutic value of herbs and alleged that they, minerals, and other objects valuable in the treatment of a particular illness could be recognized by their appropriate color or shape or by a symbol or sign they bore, a theory that came to be known as the doctrine of signatures. For example, bloodstone was good for a hemorrhage; topaz or saffron or turmeric, all yellow in hue, for jaundice; walnut meats, convoluted like the

3. All these colorful old adjectives have since disappeared from the medical books, except "venereal."
4. Allen G. Debus, *The English Paracelsians*, p. 27; John Read, *Prelude to Chemistry*, p. 27.
5. For Palmer's application of this theory, see *Admirable Secrets*, pp. 231–36.

surface of the brain, for afflictions of the head; toads covered with warts for the lesions of smallpox and syphilis; dog's liver for the bite of a mad dog. *Similia similibus curantur* went the saying: "Like things are cured by like things." Sometimes the popular name of a plant came to reflect its therapeutic use—allheal, woundwort, liverwort, heartsease, eyebright. *Admirable Secrets* contains numerous applications of the doctrine of signatures. A victim of snakebite, for example, should drink powdered Virginia snakeweed in treacle (page 69 in the original manuscript). A cough syrup should contain fox lung (page 86). It is interesting, incidentally, as Gifford points out, that some American Indian tribes also had a therapeutic rationale based on the idea that like cures like.[6]

Seventeenth-Century Medicine

In the American colonies many divines were also medical practitioners, caring for soul and body alike when members of their flocks were in trouble. A classical education served well as the foundation for advanced study in both professions. This duality of function is not new; the healer-priest is, after all, a figure of great antiquity. Not surprisingly, the equally ancient idea that illness could be the result of sin and was a punishment for it held sway among the New England settlers, who were deeply religious. About the time that Thomas Palmer completed *Admirable Secrets*, Cotton Mather (1663–1728), eminent Puritan divine and part-time medical practitioner, wrote in *The Great Physician* that "our moral distempers are the cause of our natural ones."[7] Palmer reveals the same belief in his vade mecum: "Know that Sin is the Cause of all Diseases, and sometimes

---

6. George E. Gifford, Jr., "Botanic Remedies in Colonial Massachusetts, 1620–1820," in Cash *et al.*, pp. 50, 269. Additional sources: Erwin H. Ackerknecht, *Therapeutics from the Primitives to the Twentieth Century*, p. 67; Ortho T. Beall, Jr., and Richard H. Shryock, *Cotton Mather: First Significant Figure in American Medicine*, p. 25; Malcolm S. Beinfield, "The Early New England Doctor: An Adaptation to a Provincial Environment"; Audrey Eccles, *Obstetrics and Gynaecology in Tudor and Stuart England*, pp. 18, 20; Edward Eggleston, *The Transit of Civilization*, pp. 50–57.

7. Page 6.

Diseases are immediately sent by God, and he alone must take them away by himself without instrumental means" (page 219).

The theory of humors and of the balance of natural, vital, and animal spirits; the doctrine of signatures; chemiatric medicine; the influence of miasmata, contagion, and especially the planets in their conjunctions; and belief in sickness as a form of divine retribution—all continued to be factors in seventeenth-century medicine. Understandably, when the practitioner took all these elements into consideration, therapy became a complex and sometimes risky matter.

Although Palmer cites Nicholas Culpeper (1616–54) only half a dozen times, most of Palmer's recipes are to be found in one or another of the editions of Culpeper's popular *Pharmacopeia Londinensis*, of which more later, and it is likely that the writings of the famous herbalist did much to guide Palmer's thinking and practice. Indeed, Poynter, in an authoritative study, states that historically Culpeper is "a figure of outstanding importance, for he had a far greater influence on medical practice in England between 1650 and 1750 than either Harvey or Sydenham."[8] Culpeper classified remedies into twenty-four categories according to their mode of action—emollient, hardening, attenuating, scarifying, provoking urine, and so on.[9] He also discussed medicines according to the part of the body on which they would act, enumerating those "appropriate" to the head, breast and lungs, heart, stomach, and so on.[10] He warned: "Have a care you use not such Medicines to one part of your body which are appropriate to another; for if your Brain be over-heated, and you use such medicines as cool the Heart or Liver, you make mad work."[11]

Food and drink, also important in therapy, were classified as to their degree of heat, coolness, dryness, and moistness. Seventeenth-century theory comprehended digestion as concoction—literally,

8. F. N. L. Poynter, "Nicholas Culpeper and His Books."
9. *Pharmacopoeia Londinensis*, pp. 283–98.
10. Ibid., pp. 273–83.
11. Ibid., unnumbered page.

cooking together. There were three stages in the process. Let Palmer explain:

> Humours are the excremental part or the superfluities of the first, second or third concoction . . . .
>
> 1. The first concoction is in the stomach; if the stomach be cold there is imperfect digestion, much crudities ingendred.
>
> If the Stomach be too hot, causeth much appetite, burnt & cholerick humours, much provocation to vomit, bitter tast in the mouth.
>
> 2. [The second] Concoction is in the Liver & meseraical [mesenteric] veins; the excrement of this concoction is Choler. It is sent to the Gaule [bladder] if the Gaul & the passages thereto be not obstructed. Note that the Spleen draweth away the Melancholly juice [i.e., black bile] or excrement and the kidneys, the whey or watery juice or excrement.
>
> 3. *As for the last concoction I shall better forbear saying, not willing to dwell any longer upon these matters* [page 14].[12]

According to the theory of concoction, the heat of the liver cooked the food, converting the useful part into blood. In the third concoction, which Palmer chooses not to describe, some blood was transformed into flesh and some, conveyed to various organs, was converted by them into additional substances. Thus the testes concocted blood into semen; the breasts into milk; the uterus into menses. Sweat and vapors were excreted through the skin as waste products.[13]

On page 49 Palmer enunciates an important concept in the relation of concoction to disease. "Observe by the way that ordinarily diseases begin in the Stomach and in the beginning may be easily expelled by Vomit or Siege." What are to be expelled are actually the "crudities" or imperfectly digested foods that cause disease, an idea that goes far to explain the popularity of "pukes and purges" in Palmer's day. However, if treatment of the patient is for any

---

12. Parts of *Admirable Secrets* were written in shorthand. Transcriptions of all such passages are reproduced in italics.

13. Eccles, pp. 20–21.

reason delayed, "much of the disease [from the crudities] is sucked into the Veins & then sweating Medicines is to be applyed" in order to purify the blood. Culpeper talks in some detail about sweating or "discussive" medicines (page 289).

Another concept prominent in seventeenth-century medicine had been brought forward from Greek times by Paracelsus and a few others. This idea, important in diagnosis and treatment, was that illness instead of being a poorly defined condition—fever, abdominal distress, and so on—was a manifestation of a specific disease—for example, what we would call malaria. In the seventeenth century Thomas Sydenham (1624–89) vigorously supported this view:

> In the first place, it is necessary that all diseases be reduced to definite and certain species, and that, with the same care which we see exhibited by botanists in their phytologies; since it happens, at present, that many diseases, although included in the same genus, mentioned with a common nomenclature, and resembling one another in several symptoms, are, notwithstanding, different in their natures, and require a different medical treatment.[14]

There is almost no evidence that the idea of specific diseases had reached Palmer. In general he says little about what we would call differential diagnosis, although an exception is found on page 79, where he specifies the symptoms distinguishing intestinal colic from the pain of kidney stone. However, groping toward some diagnostic specificity, he does speak at length of "presages"—signs warning of various morbid conditions and their probable outcome. For example, there were:

Presaged by Squinancys
1. Great pain, difficult breathing; no swelling appear[s] outwardly; usually kills in 4 days.
2. If a squinancy increase on a critical day, break not inwardly or outwardly, a deadly signe.

14. Thomas Sydenham, *Works*, vol. 1, p. 13.

3. If a read [red] humour appear outward & fall in again, dangerous (page 12).[15]

The patient's age and the current position of the planets also had to be taken into account.

Although residents of the New England colonies had some protection against contagious disease by virtue of the relative isolation of the settlements, deadly epidemics did occur, and other diseases were endemic. The list includes "plague . . ., measles, tuberculosis, scurvy, typhoid, dysentery, pneumonia, influenza, and yellow fever."[16] Palmer relates that in 1676 (he would then have been about ten years old), "many fell sick and died in several Towns in N. England of a putrid fever [typhus] that proved very mortal" (page 112), but he had little else to say about the incidence of various ailments.

Now let us turn briefly to the kinds of treatment available to our author and his fellow practitioners. Since illness was usually associated with an imbalance of humors, a basic purpose of therapy was to redress the balance by stimulating the increase of a deficient humor or, perhaps more commonly, by "purging" the humor that was in excess. For the latter, bleeding was frequently the procedure of choice. A migraine headache, for example, could be eased by "opening of a Vein in the forehead or nostrils" (page 127). The blood so drawn was believed to come entirely from the head.[17] Any practitioner, be he physician, surgeon, barber surgeon, leech, or charlatan,

15. Palmer's "presages" are strongly reminiscent of Hippocrates' "prognostics," reflecting the pervasive Greek influence in seventeenth-century Western medicine. For example, Hippocrates talks about ulceration of the throat associated with fever. The Greek name for this disease was translated as *quinsy*, a variant of Palmer's *squinancy*. Compare Hippocrates' statement, "Those quinsies are most dangerous, and most quickly prove fatal, which make no appearance in the fauces, nor in the neck, but occasion very great pain and difficulty of breathing; these induce suffocation on the first day, or on the second, the third, or the fourth" (Francis Adams, *The Genuine Works of Hippocrates*, 23rd Prognostic, p. 56), with Palmer's first presage by squinancies, above.

16. Gordon W. Jones, ed., *The Angel of Bethesda, by Cotton Mather*, pp. xxxi–xxxii.

17. William Harvey's proof of the circulation of the blood, although published in 1628, was still far from universally accepted at the end of the century.

was free to draw blood and did so, sometimes in alarming quantities. Blood was often let simply by opening a vein (phlebotomy). In wet cupping an incision was made, and a heated cup was tightly applied over it; the partial vacuum that developed as the cup cooled increased the flow of blood. Sometimes many small incisions were made at once with a scarificator, a handy device from which several knife tips jabbed when a spring was released. Or leeches were applied. Important considerations in bleeding included the patient's age, the location of the ailment and hence the appropriate vein to be opened, the planet that controlled the affected part of the body, and the planets then in ascendance. Anatomical knowledge was usually very slight. Palmer, for example, says that the blood in the hemorrhoidal vein comes from the spleen; bleeding from this vein is thus "profitable" (page 96).

Counterirritation, the production of a surface injury to relieve a more deep-seated ailment by purging the offending humor, was much in favor. Blisters were induced by vesicants or by dry cupping, the application of a heated cup to intact skin. Or a seton, a string or wick, could be drawn through a fold of skin to produce a fistula from which the humor could escape. Somewhat less drastic was sweating, induced by diaphoretic drugs, fomentation, poulticing, and fumigation.

In particular therapeutic favor was purging. Emetics and cathartics were numerous, were possessed of varying degrees of power, and on occasion were of remarkable complexity and cost. Sometimes purging "both upward and downward" was recommended for the wretched patient. The purpose of all this, once again, was the reduction of the peccant humors and the removal of the digestive crudities. The patient was reassured by the belief that the vile-tasting and perhaps expensive draught he had swallowed had at least acted powerfully on his behalf. Seventeenth-century medicine did not really understand how the purges worked. Culpeper addressed the problem in his usual forthright style: "Much jarring [controversy] hath been amongst Physitians about purging Medicines, namely, whether they draw the humours to them by a hidden quality, which in plain English is, they know not how; or whether they perform their office by manifest quality, *viz.* By heat, driness, coldness or moisture" (page 298).

Purges were administered internally by mouth or clyster (enema) and externally by application to the skin. It is important to recall that at this time it was believed that the active principles of many herbs could pass through the pores of the skin, find their way to a deep-seated malady—for example in the liver—and dispel a humor.[18] Alternatively, suitable "attractive" ointments or plasters, spread on the surface of a limb in which "the vital Spirit decaies . . . do not only cherish [warm, comfort] the parts, by their own proper heat, but draw the natural and vital Spirits thither, whereby they are both quickned and nourished."[19] Many recipes for oils, ointments, cerecloths, and plasters appear in the pharmacopoeias.[20]

Herbals and Pharmacopoeias

Plants are a very ancient source of medicines. Much plant lore was compiled in manuscripts and books called herbals. These described in words and pictures the habitat, appearance, qualities, and uses of plants not only for medicines but also for food, cosmetics, and other domestic purposes. The herbals seem to have been widely read during the Renaissance and later.

At the same time that herbal lore was accumulating, a vast store of folk beliefs about the curative properties of all sorts of animal preparations was developing. An extraordinary array of parts—hair, skin, fat, blood, bone, flesh, brain, organs, bile, and even excreta—from creatures as familiar as the hen, as unavailable as the elephant, and as imaginary as the unicorn were reputed to be cures, mostly infallible, for all of man's ills. The doctrine of signatures is often

18. Roger Rolls, "Bark, Blisters and the Bathe: Some Problems of Pain Relief in Former Times."

19. Culpeper, pp. 288–89.

20. Sources for the preceding section: Beall and Shryock, pp. 25–26; Beinfield, pp. 103–04; Eccles, pp. 18–21; Eggleston, pp. 50–58; Gifford, pp. 263–65. For a more extended discussion, see Allen G. Debus, ed., *Medicine in Seventeenth Century England.*

apparent; bear's grease, for example, would cure baldness, and the bone found in a deer's heart, if taken as powder, says Culpeper, "is as soveraign a Cordial, and as great a strengthener of the Heart as any is" (page 49). Medical lore was included in such early, popular compilations of information about animals as Conrad Gesner's great *Historia animalium*.

A third source of remedies were precious and semiprecious stones and a few inorganic substances such as lodestone (magnetite, or magnetized iron ore), sulphur, alum, and lead. They were employed both as charms and, ground to powder, as ingredients in various medicines. The principle that like cures like turns up again in lithotherapy, as it was called; bloodstone would stop bleeding, sapphire was cooling, and toadstone would draw out poison. Some herbals included sections on animal remedies and lithotherapy. The authors went to great pains to compile, albeit not critically, to arrange systematically, and to illustrate huge amounts of information about not only the "virtues," or curative properties, of plants, animals, and stones but also their appearance, varieties, and habitats. Such compendia helped to establish the systematic study of botany, zoology, and mineralogy and preserved for later generations a great storehouse of myth and superstition. The volumes are fascinating.

Copeman reminds us that with the growth and increasing importance of the apothecary's trade in the Tudor period, technical books of remedies called pharmacopoeias began to appear, in effect separating professional from lay works on medicine.[21] In 1618 the Royal College of Physicians of London published in Latin the first edition of its *Pharmacopoeia Londinensis*.

In that year Nicholas Culpeper, to become one of the most controversial figures in seventeenth-century English medicine, was two years old. A minister's son, he gained a good education at Cambridge but, refusing to complete the work for a degree, was placed as an apprentice to a London apothecary. Much assisted by his facility in

21. W. S. C. Copeman, *Doctors and Disease in Tudor Times*, pp. 96–97. In 1617 the London apothecaries left the Grocer's Company, which up to then had controlled the preparation and sale of drugs, to establish their own guild, the Worshipful Society of Apothecaries.

Latin, he acquired a good knowledge of *materia medica,* then turned
to medical studies, learning, like most practitioners of his day, chiefly
from books. Culpeper was never granted a university diploma. In
1640 he established a practice as a physician and astrologer.[22] He
soon had numerous patients and became noted for his special sympathy to those who were poor.

In part because of his political persuasion, outspokenness, and
biting tongue, this herbalist has been abused as a quack, but the
charge is unjustified. Culpeper's "translations of the leading European medical writers of his age gave to English doctors for the first
time a comprehensive body of medical literature in their own tongue
which represented the best contemporary authorities."[23] His numerous and very successful books were written during a brief span;
he died at the age of thirty-eight.

In 1649 Culpeper published the first translation into English of
the Royal College of Physician's *Pharmacopoeia Londinensis* and
brought down the wrath of that august body upon his head. He was
not a member of the College, and his translation was unauthorized.
However, publication of the book seems not to have been illegal,
and *A Physicall Directory,* as the first edition (1649) was called, served
the important purpose of making the contents of the *Pharmacopoeia*
available for the first time to the numerous English and colonial
medical practitioners who could not read Latin. The quarrel between
Culpeper and the College continued for years, both sides publishing
unseemly diatribes. The situation was not helped by the fact that
the doughty herbalist was a Puritan, a Parliamentarian, and a po-
pularizer locked in, and seemingly enjoying, combat with an august
and unyielding professional body under Royal charter (1518) and of
Royalist persuasion.[24]

The success of Culpeper's books continued long after his death
in 1654, both in England and the colonies. However, the first of his

22. Astrology was widely accepted at this period, not only by laymen, but by
physicians like William Harvey.

23. Poynter. p. 153.

24. Burton Chance, " 'Nicholas Culpeper, Gent: Student in Physick and Astrologie,' 1616–1653–4"; David L. Cowen, "The Boston Editions of Nicholas Culpeper"; see n. 8.

works to be published in America, *The English Physician*, did not
appear there until 1708,[25] fourteen years after *Admirable Secrets*. The
copy of Culpeper used by Thomas Palmer must have come from
London.

The content of Culpeper's *Pharmacopoeia Londinensis*, or, *The London Dispensatory*, is important to us, because his theories and many
of his recipes reappear in *Admirable Secrets*. The 1675 *Dispensatory*
begins with "An Astrologo-Physical Discourse of the Humane Vertues in the Body of Man." Here are enumerated the six human
instincts, the three kinds of spirits, the four humors, and the five
senses. Miscellaneous terms are defined. A page or so is devoted to
weights and measures. There follows "A Premonitory Epistle to the
Reader"—a kind of philosophical preface—and brief notes by the
translator.

The main portion of the book, "The Physitians Library," de-
scribes individually the curative virtues of roots, barks, and "Metals,
Stones, Salts, and other Minerals."[26] All of these are *simples*, and the
heat, coolness, wetness, or dryness of each is specified, often in
terms of degree.

There follows a long section on compounds—that is, mixtures of
two or more simples—and their medicinal virtues. The categories
are entitled Spirit and Compound Distilled Waters, Tinctures, Physical [medicinal] Wines, Physical Vinegars, Decoctions, Syrups, Rol,
or, Sapa, and Juyces, Lohoch, or, Eclegmata, Preserves, Powders,
Electuaries, Pills, Troches, Oyls, Compound Oyls, Cere-Cloaths,
Plaisters, Chymical Oils, and Chymical Preparations. Some miscellaneous directions follow. Finally, thirty-nine pages are devoted to
"A Key to Galen and Hippocrates, their Method of Physick," a
careful exposition of medical theory. Interspersed throughout the
book are Culpeper's pithy and sometimes caustic comments on "the
College's" remedies and errors, together with, he says, between two
and three hundred additions of his own (page 265). The reader's
knowledge of some medical botany is assumed.

25. See Cowen.
26. A useful index contains the additional categories of flowers, fruits and buds,
seeds, gums and rosins, juices, Living Creatures, Parts of Living Creatures, and
Belonging to the Sea (amber, pearls, spermaceti, and so on).

Palmer cites, although not frequently, the authorities on whom he depended. Sometimes he mentions a title. He does not specify years of publication; the dates included below are those of first editions unless otherwise stated. The following are the authors and sources named by Palmer, together with the pages on which they are mentioned:

Arnold, Dr. *Brevis physicae appendix*. Latin manuscript. (page 113).

Barrow (Barrough), Sir Philip. *The Method of Phisick*. (Page 111).

Boorde, Andrew. *The Breviary of Helthe*. (Page 111).

Cooke, James. (Pages 31, 49, 53, 117, 123). His two works on surgery, not specified by Palmer:

  Melleficium chirurgiae.
  Supplementum chirurgiae.

Culpeper, Nicholas. *Pharmacopoeia Londinensis*, or *The London Dispensatory*.[27] (Pages 19, 33, 34, 46, 47).

———. *The English Physitian*.[28] (Page 224).

French, John. *The Art of Distillation*. (Pages 28, 51).

Fuller, Samuel. (Title page, pages 84, 96, 210).

Galen. (Page 77).

Gerarde, John. *The Herball*. (Pages 58, 60, 223).

Hippocrates. (Page 7).

Leesens. (Page 111).

Mizaldus. (Page 245).

Riverius, Lazarius. *Riverius Reformatus*. (Page 60).

Schroderus, Johannes. *Pharmacopoeia Medico-chymica*. (Page 19).

Wirtzung, Christopher. *The General Practice of Physicke*.[29] (Pages 67, 92, 93, 95, 96).

Woodall, John. *The Surgion's Mate*. (Pages 19, 32).

Palmer also refers to a "Vade Mecum, the broad paper book with wash leather cover" (page 37) and "Vad. Mecum with Deers lether covers" (page 74), but its author is not named. Could the volume

27. See n. 2.
28. See n. 25.
29. There were editions in 16—, 1605, 1617, and 1654, brought out by various publishers.

have belonged to Dr. Samuel Fuller, his mentor, to whom Palmer acknowledges a debt on the title page of *Admirable Secrets?*[30] He also speaks of a Mr. Arch (page 27), a Dr. Butler (page 7), and a Mr. Cheney (page 89).

Admirable Secrets refers to various North American plants and animals, including moose and raccoon (page 90), and to American Indians and their remedies (pages 39, 74, 107, 149, 156, 166), one of the latter being "rock oil," or petroleum (page 41). Palmer was following the example of other colonial medical men in recognizing the medical value of native remedies. He may have been familiar with Josselyn's *New England Rarities Discovered* (1672).[31] Additional but unorthodox curative agents were the two or three charms that he mentions with some embarrassment (pages 84, 147, 240).

Some Seventeenth-Century Colonial Physicians

As we see from the title page of *Admirable Secrets*, a good part of the vade mecum was drawn from the manuscript of "Dr. Full.," identified in the text as Dr. Fuller. Who was he? There are, it seems, two possibilities. One was Thomas Fuller, M.D. (1654–1734), an Englishman who received his medical degree from Queen's College, Cambridge, in 1678. His published works include *Pharmacopoeia extemporanea* (1710) and *Pharmacopoeia domestica* (1723), which could of course have existed in manuscript form for years before they appeared in print. But Thomas Fuller, who would have been forty-two years old when *Admirable Secrets* was completed in 1696, practiced all his professional life in Sevenoaks, Kent, and there is no record that he ever visited America or had contacts there.[32] It appears most unlikely that he was Thomas Palmer's Dr. Fuller.

The other possibility is Samuel Fuller, baptized 29 January 1580

---

30. Fuller is also referred to on pp. 84, 96, 109, 123, and 210.
31. John Josselyn; Eggleston, pp. 67–68; Gifford, pp. 270–73.
32. Norman Moore, "Fuller, Thomas," in *Dictionary of National Biography*, ed. Sidney Lee, vol. 7, pp. 760–61; William Munk, *The Roll of the Royal College of Physicians of London*, vol. 1, pp. 400–01.

at Redenhall in the county of Norfolk, England, and the son of a prosperous butcher. Nothing seems to be known about his education or the nature of his medical training. "Dr." was probably a courtesy title.[33] As a youth he became a friend of William Bradford and in 1609 moved with him, William Brewster, and other Puritans to Leyden in Holland. There he lived for eleven years, active in the affairs of the congregation and appointed a deacon. Viets believes that during this period Fuller acquired a good deal of medical knowledge from William Brewster, a clergyman with a medical education.[34] Harrington affirms that "while he (Fuller) was well educated in clerical matters, his profession was medicine, and it was as a physician and not as a minister that he came to America."[35] In 1620, at the age of forty, Fuller sailed as medical attendant to the Pilgrims on *The Mayflower*. Illness and death struck almost as soon as they reached Cape Cod Harbor. Dr. Fuller was to be very busy in the ensuing months and indeed in the years to come. He made his home in Plymouth but undertook many professional visits to other settlements in the area and was widely respected for his skill. He died in a smallpox epidemic in 1633.[36]

Although definitive proof is lacking, it seems very probable that the manuscript on which Thomas Palmer drew for *Admirable Secrets* was that of Samuel Fuller. It is true that Fuller died long before 1696, the date on the vade mecum. But he could well have written a medical manuscript and left it behind in Plymouth, where Thomas Palmer was to spend most of his life. Such a document would properly have been stored with published works on medicine, and the

33. Palmer speaks three times of Dr. Fuller and twice of Mr. Fuller.
34. Henry R. Viets, *A Brief History of Medicine in Massachusetts*, p. 10.
35. Thomas F. Harrington, "Dr. Samuel Fuller of the Mayflower (1620), the pioneer physician."
36. Maurice B. Gordon, *Aesculapius Comes to the Colonies*, pp. 59–60; n. 35; Howard A. Kelly, *A Cyclopedia of American Medical Biography*, vol. 1, pp. 325–26; Francis R. Packard, *History of Medicine in the United States*, pp. 8–10; James Thacher, *American Medical Biography*, pp. 266–67; Viets, pp. 9–17; William C. Wigglesworth, "Surgery in Massachusetts, 1620–1800," in Cash et al., pp. 216–17; MacIver Woody to Janet Doe, 11 June 1953, in *Author Catalogue of the New York Academy of Medicine*, vol. 43, p. 287, item Q 10153.

latter, we know, were eagerly sought out by Palmer. It would not have been at all surprising if the Fuller manuscript, now apparently lost, had come into young Thomas's hands. Who were the *"multis aliis,"* the many other "skilfull Doctors" from whom Palmer drew his material? Most were probably the authorities he cites in *Admirable Secrets.* However, three additional medical contemporaries, although not mentioned by Palmer, may have influenced him. Like most members of the hardworking New England medical fraternity, they had occasion to travel extensively in order to see patients and must have been widely known. One was John Winthrop, Jr. (1606–76), son of the governor of Massachusetts. A student of science and law, a barrister of the Inner Temple, and a founder of the Royal Society, he came to New England in 1631 from London. Winthrop, a follower of Paracelsus's school of iatrochemistry, was medically trained like his father. During a distinguished career that culminated in several years of public service as governor of Connecticut, he found time to practice medicine in various New England towns. Winthrop had many prominent patients.[37]

Another prominent physician was Thomas Thacher (1620–78), who migrated from England as a youth. He was educated in America by Charles Chauncy, then minister of the church in Scituate, southeast of Boston, and subsequently a president of Harvard. Along with a liberal education, Thacher acquired some knowledge of medicine. Later he divided his time between the ministry, to which he was ordained, and work as a physician.[38] In 1678 he published a broadside, *A Brief Rule to guide the Common People of New England how to order themselves and theirs in the Small Pocks, or Measles.*[39] This document was the first medical work to be both written and published in

37. C. Helen Brock, "The Influence of Europe on Colonial Massachusetts Medicine," in Cash et al., pp. 101–16; Walter R. Steiner, "Governor John Winthrop, Jr., of Connecticut, as a Physician"; Herbert Thoms, *Jared Eliot, Minister, Doctor, Scientist, and His Connecticut,* pp. 13–15.

38. Viets, pp. 28–29.

39. Thacher's *Brief Rule* was dated 21.11.1677/78, which by our reckoning was 21 January 1678, given that, until 1752, New Year's Day was on 25 March.

40. Thomas Vincent's *God's Terrible Voice in the City of London,* a brief volume having to do with the plague and fire of 1665 and 1666, respectively, had been written in England.

America.[40] Since Thacher died when Palmer would have been about twelve years old, the likelihood that he knew and influenced the author of *Admirable Secrets* directly is not great.

The third unnamed contemporary who may have influenced Palmer was Cotton Mather, who succeeded Thacher as the best-known New England cleric and leading medical theorist of his day.[41] Entering Harvard at the precocious age of twelve, he undertook preparation for the ministry. However, a developing fear that his stammering would prevent him from preaching led him to take up the study of medicine, an endeavor pursued in those days mostly by reading. He earned bachelor and master of arts degrees from Harvard, became a renowned Congregational minister, and lived all his life in Boston. In addition, Mather not only kept abreast of the scientific literature but managed to publish about 450 books and articles of his own and was the first American to be elected a Fellow of the Royal Society of London. However, he never actually treated patients.[42]

In the medical area Mather is best known for his advocacy in 1721 of inoculation for smallpox and for his authorship of *The Great Physician* (1700) and *The Angel of Bethesda*. The latter, a lengthy manuscript, was completed in 1724, but no publisher could be found.[43] Exemplifying the great divine's conviction that theology and medicine are parts of the same whole, *The Angel of Bethesda*, is an admixture of religious exhortation and praise with quite temporal medical advice and recipes. Predictably, the theme was that sickness was the result of sin, and that soul and body must be cured together.[44]

Of course *Admirable Secrets* antedated this book and much else that Mather wrote, but we can speculate that Palmer, himself also a cleric-

41. Brock, p. 109.
42. Jones, p. xiv.
43. Beall and Shryock, p. 33; Brock, p. 109. Mather's great work, edited by Gordon W. Jones, was finally published by the American Antiquarian Society in 1972. The book is not to be confused with Mather's eighteen-page volume of the same name (New-London: Timothy Green, 1722); R. B. Austin, *Early American Medical Imprints 1668–1820*.
44. Beall and Shryock, pp. 9–10, 33, 53; Geoffrey Marks and William K. Beatty, *The Story of Medicine in America*, pp. 45–49; Kenneth B. Murdock, "Cotton Mather," in *Dictionary of American Biography*, ed. Dumas Malone, vol. 12, pp. 368–69.

physician, may in the last decade or so of the 1600s have fallen under the influence of the great Boston preacher.

Of the author of *Admirable Secrets* we know little. He is not to be confused with an English physician of the same name who also practiced during the latter part of the seventeeth century. Munk's *Roll*, which does not include the dates of the English Palmer's birth and death, offers no hint that the latter was also a minister or that he was ever in America. The available information about the author of the vade mecum was collected some years ago by MacIver Woody.[45] He wrote:

> Dr. Thomas Palmer, the author of *Admirable Secrets in Physick & Chyrurgery*, was born about 1666, the only son of Thomas Palmer (c. 1636–1689), mariner, of Scituate and his wife Elizabeth Russell (1642–1687/8). He died 17 June 1743, at Middleborough, Massachusetts.
>
> So far as we know, his entire life was spent within the bounds of the Plymouth Plantations. Up to 1690, and perhaps later, he lived at Scituate; he then moved to the town of Plymouth, leaving there in 1696 to accept a call to preach at Middleborough. Dissension within the local church delayed his ordination as their second minister until 1702, and in 1708 he agreed to his dismissal on the condition that he be permitted to remain and practice medicine in the community. As a physician, he was highly successful. He raised a large family, put two sons through Harvard, and left an estate valued at £7176:06:03, of which £948:06:03 was personal goods, including books.[46]

Notes in the hands of Thomas Palmer and others on the back flyleaf of *Admirable Secrets* indicate that his mother, Elizabeth, died 1 February 1688 at age 44, and that his father, Thomas, succumbed in Port Royal, Jamaica, on 16 June 1689, aged either forty (shorthand entry) or fifty years (longhand entry). The latter seems more plau-

---

45. Dr. Woody, then of Elizabeth, N.J., and a direct descendant of Palmer, had long been a student of *Admirable Secrets* and had searched extensively for biographical details about its author (Mrs. Woody to Thomas Rogers Forbes, 8 January 1978).

46. MacIver Woody to Janet Doe, 11 June 1953. Quotation by courtesy of Mrs. Woody and the New York Academy of Medicine Library.

sible. Thomas Palmer the younger, author of *Admirable Secrets*, died, as we know, on 17 June 1743. His wife, named Elizabeth like his mother, died 16 April 1740, aged about sixty-four. As to their offspring, Palmer mentions only "one of my children" (page 203).[47] In combining medicine and the ministry, he was, of course, following a well-established tradition. Since there is no record that Palmer ever left America, and since the colonies did not yet have a medical school, his medical knowledge, like that of most of his contemporaries, must have been acquired through reading and possibly, although there is no direct evidence for this, from an apprenticeship. The vade mecum reveals little understanding of anatomy or chemistry. However, Palmer's knowledge of physic was considerable and orthodox. He understood the theory of humors, the doctrine of signatures, Paracelsian principles of medicine, and the process of concoction, and their rational application in diagnosis and treatment. He gave some attention, as did his contemporaries, to medical astrology and was familiar with medical botany. His faith in the efficacy of his remedies—*probatum est* was his highest praise—may seem excessive, but the remedies had the support of authority and experience, and he knew nothing more effective.

The title of the manuscript promises the reader the best of both medicine and surgery, but there is relatively little of the latter. One reason is that the author probably never dissected a human body; he may never even have witnessed a dissection. Also, surgery is not to be learned just from books; if Palmer, as seems likely, had seen little surgery done by others, he would be understandably hesitant to attempt it himself. An exception to this generalization is his interesting and realistic description of the treatment of fistula (pages 114–15). It is obvious, however, that he preferred the conservative, nonsurgical treatment of such problems as hernia and hydrocele (pages 134–39). Finally, we find in *Admirable Secrets* no mention of the care and delivery of pregnant women; clearly Palmer, like most of his contemporaries, left this to the midwives.

In Palmer's discourse on "The Reason why many fall short of the Benefits of Medicine" (page 219) we can discern some of his own

47. Perhaps this was Mary Palmer, great-great-great-grandmother of Mrs. Regina Woody (Woody to Forbes, 8 January 1978).

guiding principles. Physicians, he says, may sometimes fail to cure their patients because the latter are uncooperative or unreasonable or unwilling to pay for treatment. But medical men also fail when they forget that sin is the cause of disease, and that sickness ultimately is cured by God. No doctor should be wicked or greedy or unwise or promise that which he cannot perform. In particular no healer should be lacking in knowledge, failing to understand nature and how to help her. Wisdom comes from reading. "But how few have the knowledge of the secret mysteries of physick? I have seen and read many authors," he says proudly, "the best part of 30."

Here is Thomas Palmer the young physician, relying on his books, on experience, and on the dicta of other, more experienced heads, committed to a simple but admirable code of conduct, supported by his faith in God. Stalwart against the harsh background of the early New England settlements, he stands independently in unremitting daily conflict with sickness, trusting to humoral theory and strange herbal mixtures. Judged against the context of his time, he has our respect.

Admirable Secrets

Only three medical books were published in the colonies before 1696. Thomas Vincent's *God's Terrible Voice in the City of London* of 1668 described London's plague and fire in 1665 and 1666, respectively, and reviewed the resulting bills of mortality. Thomas Thacher's *A Brief Rule* appeared in 1678 and was followed by John Oliver's *A Present To Be Given to Teeming Women* (1694), a book on midwifery. To the list might be added Cotton Mather's *Memorable Providences* and *Balsamum vulnerarium*, which, although not medical in their intent, did consider some forms of mental illness.[48] Palmer, incidentally, cited none of these books.

In 1643 a Dr. Edward Stafford of London had written a manuscript

48. Austin, pp. 152, 199, 204, 225; Francisco Guerra, *American Medical Biography 1639–1783*, pp. 29–32; Richard H. Shryock, *Medicine and Society in America 1660–1860*, p. 47.

of eight and a half pages called "Receipts to Cure Various Disorders," addressing it to "my worthy friend Mr. Winthrop," who may have been John Winthrop, Sr., or John Winthrop, Jr. The document recited remedies for seventeen illnesses and injuries, together with a list of "Cautions in Physick." Although drafted in England, it was produced for colonial consumption and may have been the first unpublished compilation of its kind to be used on this side of the Atlantic.[49] Edward Taylor (1642–1729), a Connecticut minister and poet, was the author of an undated manuscript entitled "Dispensatory," which, says Leighton, gives the names and virtues of almost four hundred plants.[50]

Among all these *Admirable Secrets* stands alone, of unique importance in seventeenth-century colonial medical history. Palmer uses the word *secrets* in the Elizabethan sense, referring to specific and infallible remedies. Here are his diagnostic signs and what they foretold—the presages—and here are the secrets on which the medical man chiefly depended. Palmer preserves for us in his simple way a careful record, an epitome of the elements of medical theory and practice as they were understood. The sentence structure and style strongly suggest that the little book was meant for his own use; only once does he refer to a "friendly Reader" (page 218). He tells it all in a single notebook. Unlike the weighty printed volumes that must remain on his or his friends' shelves, his vade mecum could be slipped into saddlebag or coat pocket, and he could then hurry forth, armed for attack on the impatient enemy. Sometimes, as Palmer grimly remarked, "Death comes galloping" (page 9).

Strangely enough, the whereabouts of the original of *Admirable Secrets* is unknown. My letters or visits to twenty-four leading libraries in the United States and London and my search in numerous catalogues of manuscripts have thus far uncovered no clues as to the location of the missing notebook. There is a photocopy of *Admirable Secrets* at the Countway Library and another at the Library of the Massachusetts Historical Society, and the Library of the New York

49. Gordon, pp. 63–67; Oliver Wendell Holmes, *Medical Essays, 1842–1882*, pp. 330–31; Packard, pp. 10–15.
50. Ann Leighton, *Early American Gardens*, pp. 115–16.

Academy of Medicine has both a photocopy and a microfilm.[51] Library catalogues indicate Middleboro, Massachusetts, as the apparent place of origin of the manuscript, but the location of the original volume and the provenance of the various copies are not recorded. The photocopy begins with the title page of *Admirable Secrets*. There follows a torn fragment; what little text it preserves suggests that at least one page preceded the damaged sheet. An unnumbered page of text is succeeded by "General Rules to be Observed . . . ," marked as page one by Palmer. Successive pages are numbered to 245 in Palmer's hand; of these, nineteen are missing from the photocopy, presumably because they were blank. Individual sheets as photographed measure 88 by 147 millimeters. The small handwriting, which suggests photographic reduction from the original, is reasonably clear, but foxing at the edges of some pages obscures words, sometimes to the point of illegibility.

In editing the manuscript, misspellings were retained. Punctuation was silently corrected only as necessary to make the meaning clear. Contractions such as *ye, wch, yn*, and *wn* were expanded to *the, which, then* or *than*, and *when*. Apothecary's symbols for weight and measure were changed to the more familiar English abbreviations. The alchemical sign ♆ , which in other sources signifies coral, manganese ore, *libra* (pound), or *calx viva* (quicklime), in Palmer's context seems to mean infusion and has been so transcribed.

Palmer's Shorthand

Some puzzling passages, usually brief, were written in what was eventually discovered to be a very early form of phonetic shorthand. Whether the author resorted to this for convenience or to protect the confidentiality of certain details is not clear. In the transcription that follows, all such passages are spelled out and printed in italics.

Systems of shorthand were known to the Romans in the first century B.C. but were subsequently almost forgotten. The early meth-

---

51. Richard J. Wolfe to Forbes, 21 December 1977 and 16 December 1981; John D. Cushing to Forbes, 9 April 1979; Inge Dupont to Forbes, 6 January 1982.

ods depended on signs to represent individual letters and some words. Modern shorthand was invented by Timothy Bright, M.D. (1551?–1615).[52] John Willis is said to have developed in 1602 the first phonetic system—that is, one in which a symbol represents the sound of a letter or combination of letters. About 1690 William Addy published his *Stenographia or the Art of Short-Writing* (1690?), which appears to have been the first book in English on phonetic shorthand. Addy's system was a modification of the systems of his seventeenth-century predecessors. The shorthand method used by Thomas Palmer resembles in part that of Addy and indeed may have been derived and modified from the latter's *Stenographia*.

At first, it seemed that it would be impossible to decode Palmer's shorthand, but a breakthrough occurred when lines that were a mixture of plain text and symbols were found on page 16. One sentence, part of some instructions on phlebotomy, read:

The Veins in the arm opened are Cephalica ⟨symbols⟩ : Basilica or ⟨symbols⟩ : Mediana ⟨symbols⟩ / ve ·|· / 2 ⟨symbols⟩. Now in the human arm the *vena cephalica* and *vena basilica* lie just under the skin and are an obvious target in bloodletting. *Vena cephalica* may be translated "head vein," so let us assume that the three groups of symbols following *Cephalica* mean *or head vein*. If so, one has meanings for six symbols and a start on the next phrase,"Basilica or ⟨symbols⟩." If the arm is held extended from the shoulder, thumb up, the basilic vein does lie lower than the cephalic. Therefore might the phrase read "Basilica or *lower vein*"? This turns out to be correct, and two more symbols have disclosed their meaning.

On the basis of what has now been learned, the third phrase could be partly decoded as follows: "Mediana *or* / *vein* ·|· / 2 ⟨symbols⟩." *The* would fit as a meaning for /, but what about the rest? Again some anatomical information is useful. In the human arm the median cubital vein connects the cephalic and basilic veins near the elbow. After further struggle, the phrase is found to read, "Mediana *or the vein*

---

52. *Characterie. An Arte of Shorte, Swifte, and Secrete Writing by Character.* The author is not to be confused with Richard Bright, M.D. (1789–1858), who described the kidney disease later named for him.

Phlebotomy or Blood-letting.

The veins in y[e] arm opened are
Cephalica. a 90 ve: Basilica or
uve ve: Mediana, a [?] ve 1. 12 [?]
The mediana is formed of y[e] branches of Cephalica & Basilica, running w[i]th in one.
[?] i ve i — [?] [?] 5 1. 1 co — 2: Cephalica
[?] — [?] Artery nor sinew near it. y[e] Mediana
hath a sinew just under it. Basilica hath with Artery and
sinew just under it. Note y[e] Cephalica sometimes w[i]th not
appear, & so sometimes [?] of y[e] other veins, and
sometimes neither of them.

In some cases blood-letting saves life, and in some
cases destroys it. y[e] abundance of blood & inflammation
of blood open a vein.

If in y[e] morning about break of day a person
useth to sweat, it argues superfluities in y[e] blood.
Abundance of blood is known by thickness & troubled
consistency of y[e] veins. Note y[e] whore [?] and
cold blood [?] [?] ought to go before.

Gul[?] [?] veins under y[e] tongue are opened for y[e]
squinancy & difficult swallowing [?] they are both
of them apparent ordinarily, when y[e] under of y[e]
tongue is turned upward — [?] [?] [?] [?] [?]
[?] [?] [?] [?] — ve co — 2 [?] [?]
2 [?] [?] so y[e] [?] 4[?] [?] squa 5 [?]
[?] & y[e] [?] y[e] [?] [?] [?] [?] near y[e]
[?] [?] & [?] y[e] [?] — [?] [?] [?]
The veins below y[e] inside of y[e] ankle [?]
[?] & women tied to be greased to help [?]
1. [?]: 1[?] [?] [?] [?] [?] [?] [?] [?] 5 [?]
5 1 [?]: if you find difficulty in stopping
y[e] blood [?] [?] wool in & blood & [?]
[?] [?] col[?] [?] [?] [?] [?] [?] [?] — [?]:
[?] [?] [?] [?] blood via a dropsy except

...Plague to any... ... ...
...poor... any humour appears. yet ... ...
blooding at ye first, provided it be at ye time of the
next blooding, to divert ye blood another way.
...

Letting of blood is often profitable for those yt have
any sore bruise in any part, to divert ye humours another
way, from flowing to the grieved bruise, as ... ...
... ... yet it ... ... need be presently as
soon as may be, before ye blood be settled congealed
or putrified ! ... ...

~ A Cerot. a Salve for Aches & Strains
for... ... ...
R a Quart of Allot Oyl a pound of...
two thirds red & one white. First ... of ...
to quarter of a pound a quant of Oyl & boyl them
together & then add ye Lead as before & boyle
together to a Salve. ... add a shilling in Saffron
Nutmeg, Mace at ... ana Egg. boyl them
in to mix them. ... little, as a shilling of oyl of
Spike add to it: you add ye Spice, boyl it in a great
skillet, for any great bruise in Bad Back or otherwise

~ Consumption in ye Lungs. for Cough.
R Feabious roots, Elecampane roots, Liquorice
Parsly roots, marigold flours, Maiden-hair
Hysop, Sage, Anniseed Horehound, Colts foot
sweet marjoram figgs, raisons in ye Sun
make a decoction in fair water, ... Syr. S. A

between the 2 former." (Only belatedly was it realized that 2 was not an arcane symbol but an Arabic numeral.)

A second helpful passage was found on page 98. Part of the sentence read:

Hydromel, i.e., ⅋⌐ ⅃↵· ꝗ—·ꝗ/ ∣–∣ɣɔ. Now, hydromel was a soothing laxative liquid made by heating honey and water together, a fact that justified several guesses. The symbol / stood for *th*; could it also stand for *t?* The symbol ↵ meant *r;* — meant *n*; ꝗ, *h*; ɔ , *d*. After substituting these sounds and experimenting further, the phrase was decoded to read, "Hydromel, i.e., *water wherein honey hath been boiled.*"

Here is a list of Palmer's symbols and of sounds they represent:

∣ b, p	⌃ k	ꝗ h, kw
↖ m	∩ k	ꝱ g (get)
╱ t, th	c b, p, k, o	⅂ ing
7 f	ɔ d	ꙅ s
∏ g (purge)	o p, uh	⅁ w, p
— n, a	e e, a	ɦ wh
ɣ ay	∨ v, w	ꝗ ch, sh
↵r	∪ l, u	

It will be noted that some symbols have two or more meanings, and that a few sounds—for example *p*—may be represented by more than one symbol. Vowel sounds, commonly omitted, could be indicated by an irregularly placed dot. In some frequently used words the symbols might be run together: *z*, composed of 7 and ∨ , meant *for;* ↳ —that is, ╱⌐ ɔ —signified *third;* 7 ꙅ —that is, 7↵ꙅ∣ —meant *first.* In a few cases the meaning of a group of symbols was ambiguous: ⟋⌐ could have been 7↵↖, *firm* or *form*, but the context showed that — ∨ ↖ , *arm*, was meant. Such short cuts did nothing to facilitate the decoding of the shorthand.

Other problems arose when symbols were carelessly or even incorrectly written. Palmer's notes, jotted down quickly for his own use, were often telegraphic in style. Finally, I had to learn to anticipate the occasional appearance in shorthand of words now archaic or obsolete—*cholered, squinancy, quartern,* and *cloddered.*

The Glossary

In the early years of the colonies textbooks of medicine, most sur-
gical instruments, and many drugs had to be imported from Europe.[53] Simples were grown in the gardens of medical practitioners,
along with kitchen spices and native fruits and vegetables for the
table. The Worshipful Society of Apothecaries had established its
own Physic Garden in Chelsea in 1673. The tradition for domestic
production of healing plants, like some of the plants themselves,
was transplanted from England. In addition, colonial practitioners
collected useful wild plants wherever they could be found in fields
and forests. For this some knowledge of medical botany was essential, and the herbals of Turner,[54] Gerarde, and others must have
been invaluable.

Complete identification of many of the plants named by Palmer
has not been possible. Our present-day binomial system for scientific
names, which was established by Linnaeus (1707–78), came after
Palmer's time. It was not unusual for the same common name to be
used for two or more quite different plants. Some generic, or family,
and specific, or individual, scientific names have been changed by
the taxonomists since Palmer used them. It is said that English popular names were sometimes incorrectly applied to American plants
they resembled, and it is likely that a few imported herbs were
hybridized with their relatives on this side of the Atlantic.[55] So iden-
tifications in the glossary have been made cautiously, and usually
any effort to designate a species has been omitted. The adjective
officinalis that occasionally appears, incidentally, identifies within a
genus a particular species approved by pharmacopoeias for official
use.

The works of reference most helpful in preparing the glossary were
Culpeper's *Pharmacopoeia Londinensis* and Dunglison's *A Dictionary
of Medical Science*. Although the latter appeared almost two centuries
after *Admirable Secrets*, such was the slow advance of medicine that

53. Brock, p. 107.
54. William Turner, *A New Herball*.
55. Eggleston, pp. 67–68; Poynter, pp. 157–58.

a great many of Palmer's terms could be found in the *Dictionary*. Other helpful works were Wirtzung's (Wirsung's) little known *The General Practice of Physicke*, translated by Jacob Mosan, and Woodall's *The Surgion's Mate*. Valuable modern sources included J. W. Estes's article on colonial therapeutic practice, Charlotte Erichsen-Brown's *Use of Plants for the Past 500 Years*, *Gray's Manual of Botany*,[56] Hans Flück's *Medicinal Plants*, B. C. Harris's *The Compleat Herbal*, and Richard Le Strange's *A History of Herbal Plants*. The ingredients in Palmer's many recipes are sometimes enumerated in the glossary; in other cases the complexity of certain compounds, containing in extreme cases up to fifty or sixty simples, made full identification impractical.

As would be expected, a good many of the medical terms are now obscure or have a different meaning. These words are explained parenthetically or in the glossary. The catchwords in the latter are as Palmer spelled them, even when incorrectly. His original page numbers have been retained. The appearance of a number in square brackets marks the beginning of the corresponding page.

56. Merritt L. Fernald, ed.

THE ADMIRABLE SECRETS
OF PHYSICK AND CHYRURGERY

Admirable Secrets in
Physick & Chyrurgery.
Transcribed
Ex Manuscripto D: Full:
Cum multis aliis, being
The Secret Practise of many Skilfull
Doctors.

Thomas Palmer
Ejus Liber:
Anno Dom:
1696

Vade Mecum.
Exod 30. 35.

Felix qui potuit rerum cognoscere causas.
Quas; timor, Surorum Saevum curabit.

And Thou shalt make it a perfume a
Confection, after y art of y Apothecary
tempered together. Exod 30. 34. 35.

Principiis obsta, sero medicina paratur,
Cum mala per longas invaluere moras.

Admirable Secrets in Physick & Chyrurgery

Transcribed
Ex Manuscripto D: Full:
Cum multis aliis being

The Secret Practise of many skilfull Doctors

Thomas Palmer
Ejus Liber
Anno Dom
1696

Vademecum
Exod. 30. 35

And thou shalt make it a perfume, a
Confection, after ye art of ye Apothecary
tempered together. Exod. 30. 34–35

Principiis obsta, sero medicina paratur,
Cum mala per longas invaluere moras.

Foelix qui potuit reru cognoscere Causas

Inque domus Superum Scandere cura fuit.

Note on the Title Page

Ex manuscripto D. Full. Cum multis aliis . . . . From the manuscript of Dr. Fuller, with many others. Ejus Liber Anno Dom[ini] 1696, His book, the Year of our Lord 1696. Principiis obsta sero medicina paratur/Cum mala per longas invaluere moras. This quote is from Ovid's *Remedia amoris* (Remedies of Love) 91–92. A suggested translation is: Resist the first advance (onset), for medicine comes late/When evils have gained strength through long delays.

Foelix qui potuit reru[m] cognoscere Causas, Fortunate is he who can understand the causes of things. This is a quotation from Virgil's *Georgics* 2.490.

Inque domus Superum Scandere cura fuit. This is a misquotation of the second line of a couplet from Ovid's *Fasti* 1.298: felices animae, quibus haec cognoscere primus/inque domus superas scandere cura fuit! (O happy souls, who first took thought to know these things and to ascend to the dwellings of the gods!)

[Unnumbered page] I once knew a certain Scholar (said Dr. *Fuller*) (illegible) *son affirmed to me that his father* drew out of fair Conduit *water* a Spirit at 3 times distilling that had the tast of low wines, as Distillers call it; the use & right improvement of it would be of very great use for medicine. Oh Lord! how wonderfull are thy Works sought out of all that have pleasure in them.

Make a strong tincture of any herb, filtre it. Make a strong Lixivium of Tarter and add to it. It will seperate the gummy substances, as wines poured into milk will seperate the Curds. It will doe of Wormwood, Rue, Carduus or any herb of strong tast. It will be like aloes bitter & brittle.

Rx. Aloes, Myrrh, Saffron, add salt of Tartar to it and spirit of wine aromatised, Distill it; that will make it yeild its Tincture. Elixir proprietatis.

Salt of Tartar, spirit of wine, usefull to make the balsamick medicine.

Mix salt & oyl till they in length of time are brought into a body. Ad spirit of wine aromatized. Distill it. This is a balsamick medicine. A Quintessence as some call it. Take your fixed salt & add it to proper distilled water. Digest it in the heat of a bath. Vapourizing the water, melt the salt in a Crucible, add it to the same water, vapour it away several times. Then mix the salt and proper oyl together. When its a body, add spirit of wine aromatised. This is the Balsam Samech. [Page 1]

General Rules to be Observed
by Those that are called to practice Physick

Whensoever thou art called to them that are sick, mind these following particulars:

1. Enquire the time they have been sick; the maner of taking,[1] and what is conceived to be the cause. Observe also the Climate & Season.

1. Onset of illness.

2. What the State & Condition of the body is, & hath been, that so thou mayst help, or further nature in the accustomed evacuations, if the part be capable & it be safe.
3. View & observe if there be any apparent signs, or many apparent signs of Death at hand: And then be sure [to] forbare [from] any working Physick, lest the patient dy within a short time after giving of the same, or nature be so spent it will not work at all.
4. Consider whether it be a humoural Distemper & what Humours are most afflictive, & what parts of the body are most distempered, & where the seat of the disease lyes, and what method must be observed in the removing of it. Some of these are found out by discoursing with the patients or those that attend them. Some are found out by much & long reading of many authours concerning signs & causes of Disseases. Some are found out by the carefull practice & experience & observation of the Physitians.

Signs of Death or Life

Presages by the Face. A good sign in Sickness, if it look in sickness as it was in health [Page 2] or little differing. It is bad to see the nose extenuated (reduced), sharp, the Eyes hollow, skin of the forehead or eyebrows hard and look a stand (askance). Ears cold, shrunk almost double, face black, pale, swarthy, deformed, when you see these be not rash but inquire whether the party have not fasted much, wanted Sleep, or had a Flux a long time.[2] If the Sickness have been four or 5 dayes before you see these Symptoms, a sign Death follows at the heels.

Presages by the Eyes & Lips

1. If deprived of Sight, or weep against the patient's will.
2. If they seem as if they would fall out of the head.
3. When one Eye is less than the other.
4. When the white of the Eye becomes reddish.
5. When they are blare [blear] eyed [but] not so before, or dim.

2. That is, are these alarming symptoms due to hunger, exhaustion, and diarrhea or to the disease itself?

6. Moveable, staring up & down as though fright'd or sunk deep in the head; squint eyed [but] not so before; stare as though frighted.
7. Sleep with the eyes open, not so before, then inquire if this came not by a Flux or laxitive in medicine, if not signs of Death. Eyelids, nose, and lips are crooked or drawn in to one side. Lips thin, cold, pale, hanging doun & the nose very sharp, it denotes death.

Presages by the manner of lying in the Bed. It is best when they lye in the same for that they did in health.

Bad Signs

1. When the neck, hands, feet are extended, stiff, and inflexible, not to be moved.
2. Sudden starting out of Bed. [Page 3]
3. Casting the Head doun to the Feet of the Bed. Sleeping with the mouth open; restless, tumbling up & down the bed; sleeping with the belly downward, not as before, shew aches of the belly little less than madness, desiring to go out of one room to another. He that is impatient and would rise upon a critical day, puts himself in great danger; if the disease be violent & touch his langurs, the critical day may prove mortal.

Presages by the Teeth

1. Gnashing the teeth in a Fever, a dangerous sign if he did not so at other times.
2. If he be deprived of his Sences, his Sicknes only a Feavour, not a frenzy, gnashing of the teeth, Death will come.

Presages by Ulcers and Issues

If they come before they are with a feavour, if they drie up & become green & black & swarthy, Death to be expected if he do not grow better.

Presages by the Hands

If in Fevers or any acute dissease, phrensie only excepted, the Sick be pidling & pulling of the bed-clothes: or catching in the ayr as tho he say something, if he had take violent hold of ye bed-clothes, seiling (ceiling) or wall these are dangerous signs.

Presages by the Breath

[1.] By the Breath is best judgment given [Page 4] upon the Spirit heart & lungs, when the disease seases (seizes) the Spirits there is no digestion found: a gentle breath in hot diseases an aug(ury) of death.

2. Distance too long between breaths & coldnes shews death.

Presages by Sweat

1. A kind Sweat that is upon a Critical or judicial day is good.
2. Mortal sweats are first of all cold & in some part only: usually if other parts do not sweat the sickness will be long.

Presages by Tumours

1. If the party sick of a Feavour feeleth neither pain, inflammation, tumour, nor hardness upon or near about his ribs, it is a good sign.
2. If any of these be there, & upon both sides, a bad sign.
3. If he feels great motion & pulsations in one of his sides, it prognosticates great pain & deprivation of his senses.
4. And if with his pulsation his eyes move faster than they should do he is in danger to fall into a phrensy or else to mischief (injure) himself.

Presages by Apostumes

1. Apostumes in a burning fever on both sides are bad.
2. Worst in the left side.
3. If it continues 20 dayes & the fever ceases not, & the impostumes diminish not it will come to maturation.
4. If a flux of blood at the nose [occurs] upon a crit(ical) day it easeth the patient: he will be pained in the head, have dim sight at noonday if under 35 years of age.
5. When the Impostume is soft & with pain, when it is handled a long time, hard to cure but not dangerous. [Page 5]

6. It may continue two months before it ripens.
7. That Impostume that is hard, great and painfull, if it be not mortal, it is dangerous.
8. Apostumes of the belly are never so great as they that grow under the Midriff, & those that grow under the navil and then they usually come to maturation.
9. It is a good sign when they purge by a flux of blood by the nose.
10. Some purge only outwardly & they are little round & sharp pointed; they are good.
11. Such as are large gross and not round, but flat are most dangerous.
12. Those that purge and breake within the belly and make Tumours outward are pernicious.
13. If that which comes out of Apostumes be white, and not unsavoury [foul smelling] it is good.
14. The more the colour differs from white the worse it is.

Presages for Dropseys in Fevers

1. Dropseys are of cold: fevers of heat. That which is given to one encreases the other.[3]
2. If a Fever & a Dropsey meet together they will play reeks, as seldom it is,[4] and then the Liver pays the Score.
3. It afflicts the Vena inschiary (ischiadica), most commonly the gutt; the legs are tormented; a flux follows; the swelling in the belly is not lessened.
4. If the liver is most afflicted, a drye Cough attends, he spits little, his belly is very hard, he goes to stoole with pain; the feet swell; there is tumour and inflammation in his side: some times they dissipate & swell again.

Presages of Life and Death In Fevers

[1.] Cold on the head and face. Cold sweats. Heands and feet cold: belly & sides hot & burning, a [Page 6] sign of Death.

3. If a dropsy is treated with heat, the fever is made worse; if a fever is treated with cold, the dropsy increases.
4. . . . play reeks, as seldom it is—that is, play pranks, which seldom happens.

2. When all the parts of the body are equally hot in a fever, tho they be hotter than ordinary it is a good sign.
3. The body heavy, the nails of a leady swarthy colour, the dissease will be cured by Death.
4. Enduring sickness without anguish, shows strength of nature.
5. Enquire after the State of the Sick when he was in health: and if his spittle, sleep, excrements be as they were when the body was in health, Health is a coming: by those signs you may know in some measure what part of the body was afflicted, & by what removed.

Presages by the Testicles

When the yard & testicles are shrunk in and apparently diminished, it signifies great pain, anguish & Death.

Presages by Sleeping

1. Sleeping in the night, & waking in the day a good sign.
2. For the sick to sleep from break of the day to 8: or 9: in the morning is the best time of day to sleep in.
3. Continual watching is extream dangerous.

Presages of Excrements of the Belly in Fevers

1. It is a good sign when he that is in a Fever hath the same coustume (custom) of avoiding his Excrements as when he was in health.
2. Mind the kind & quantity of diet, and how they differ from this, so much the worse. [Page 7]
3. Laudable Excrements, neither too thick nor too thin; Costiveness not to be allowed of.
4. Looseness in a feaver doth proclaime to the world the patient hath kept a bad diet before. It is exceeding good the Excrements be near the colour of the food taken. It is good the patient go to stoole without pain. If nature be troubled to expell the Excrements, she will find a harder pull to dispell the disease.
5. If the man sick of a fever have a looseness, & what comes from him comes with Violence, pain or wind it's a hopefull sign.

6. Yet frequent going to Stools weakens the body, & spoils digestion, Marry, the retentive faculty makes the Sick froward (cross, peevish) & faint.
7. Worms coming out of the body with the Excrements at the end of the malady is good, at the beginning of the sickness is dangerous.
8. It is good in every sickness when the belly is soft, & not puft up with wind.
9. Excrements very watery white, or very red, or froathy very dangerous, not always mortal.
10. Black green or slimy Exc[rements]: sign of Death.
11. The mixture of the forenamed Cold and dangerous.
12. Little skins like the pealing of the gutts. Mr. Culpeper's son *was failing with this disease and he before life was still was cured with blue boiling* mallows in his drink.

Presages by Wind in the Bowells

1. Wind issuing out gently & voluntarily is the best & holsomest sign.
2. Worst of all when it is retained & comes not out; bad when it comes with pain & griping. Swelling of wind in the Belly according to Hypocrates is best cured by Expulsion downwards or by Urine. Dr. Butler[5] cured a man in this case by rowling (roiling, agitating) his belly with a rowling Drink. [Page 8]

Presages by Urine in Fevers

1. Urine with white settlings in the bottom in a fever or any other disease, like a Piramid, is a good sign.
2. The more it differs from this the worse it is.
3. Gross Resolutions like dust or bran in the bottom is a bad sign, worse when they are like scales of fish.
4. Urine white & clear signifies melancholy, & that is very bad because it retains it: *it* has *not* as well as that it should.[6]

5. Not further identified.
6. A word is omitted. The author means, ". . . it (melancholy) has not disappeared as well as that it should." This is humoral medicine.

5. A white cloud hanging in the urine signifies health; if black it is dangerous.
6. Urine yellow, very clear & subtile shows crudity & indigestion.
7. In such a case there is fear lest the sick die before the humour come to concoction.[7]
8. Slimy, muddly, black, dirty, filthy, stincking urine is usually mortal.
9. A child's urine pale & clear like Cunduit [conduit] water is very bad. It signifies cold & dry [humours] but hot & most [moist] is proper to youth.
10. A thing like a Cob-web swimming on the top a bad sign.
11. Thick urine signifies a Consumption; white Clouds in the urine near the bottom are commendable; black & near the top are bad.
12. In all these have regard to the blather [bladder], for if it have disease all these presages be in vain.
13. If in a feaver the Urine appear like the Urine of a healthy man a dangerous signe. The dissease workes upon the Spirits, not the body.[8]
14. Look right under the cloud by holding the urine high, and in the lower side of the cloud appears small bright shining bubbles like small pins heads. [This] shows running pains in the limbs. [Page 9]
15. Observe in the body of the urine either shaken or not shaken small round contents, smaller than pins heads and a great many of them; [this signifies] pains in the Limbs or gouty pains.

Presages of Vomiting in Feavers

1. To Vomit up Phlegm & choler in a Fever a good sign.
2. If what be Vomited be green, livid, or black is dangerous.
3. If what be Vomited be compounded of these, its mortal.

---

7. That is, before the humor undergoes maturation or change, a necessary preliminary to its elimination. If the dangerous humour is not eliminated, the patient will die.
8. That is, the disease affects the patient's spirits.

4. If it stink that you cannot endure to hold your nose over it & have but one of these, Death comes galloping.

Presage by Spittle in Fevers

1. In all diseases of the Lungs & malady's under the ribs if it (spittle) be in the beginning of a disease, & without pain of a good colour, viscous, well digested, a good sign.
2. When the Spittle comes up with Vehement Coughing, a bad sign.
3. In a Fever white spittle, tough & knotty, a bad signe.
4. Green & fleshy spittle bad.
5. Black spittle worse, then grim death a coming.
6. When the matter that should be spitt out still remains within the lungs & troubles the wind pipe it is bad; if pain be eased by spitting it is a good sign. Black spitting & paine eased, is not so dangerous.

Presages by Sneezing In a Fever

1. Sneezing in a hot malady a good sign.
2. If Malady's in the lungs, if it be with much [Page 10] Rhume & pain felt after, it is dangerous.

Presages of Suppuration in Aposthumes

1. If the pain of an Imposthume cease not by spitting to which add laxative medicines & letting of blood, its like to come to suppuration.
2. When the Aposthume breaketh, the Spittle giving Notice of choler, whether matter comes out with the Spittle or after it is dangerous.
3. If the matter comes upon the first crisis, it comes to tell you Death will come upon the second crisis.

Presages by the time of the Rupture of Aposthems

Coughing, spitting, spauling [salivating], pain, difficulty of breathing are true signs it is near breaking. Note that the beginning of the disease, when the patient feels heat, a fever, stifnes, pain, pricking, or anything else, that denotes a disease. If that comes out Aposthems be white, equal [uniform], salt, & come out without pain, and the patient falls to his Victuals, a good sign. If the fever will return again, the thirst remains still & when the fever doth return the Feces being very watery, green, livid, or shiny, death's not far. If the patient feel pain on both sides [and] both sides are Aposthemated, cause him [to] ly on the side [that] hath less pain & if he feele heavines there its a sure sign the Aposth.[9] If some good sign & some bad appeare, compare them all-together & judge by most testimony make use of all the rules you can so you may find *truth*.

Presages of Aposthems about the Eares

When under or about the eare come to maturation and breake, the bitterness of Death is past.

SIGNS OF APOSTHUME

There is swelling, pain, heat & burning, rednes of [Page 11] colour, inflammation about the place.

APOSTHEM IN THE FEET

1. In vehement and dangerous diseases of the Lungs, it conduceth much to the help of the patient when sweat pushes or Aposth[em] appear in the feet.
2. If the Spittle change from redd to white, a good sign.
3. If it do not, the pain ceaseth not & the sinews of part Aposthemated are in danger of shrinking.
4. If together with the former the Aposthem also vanish away, the man looseth (loseth) his sences first, & his life afterwards.
5. Aged people are most subject to diseases of the Lungs.
6. Its dangerous in all Aposthems when the pain ascends upwards.
7. Easy spitting, white, & not stincking, good. Red or black stincking spittle is deadly.

Presages by the Bladder in Fevers

Hardnes, pain, stopping of urine in quotidian fever foredestines Death. In aposthems of the Bladder when they come to scurvie

9. Remainder of sentence was omitted.

places, if the urine & like matter of the Aposthem and the paine ceases & fever mitigated & the Bladder mollified, those signs argue the worst to be past. This disease usually happeneth to few but children & to them most usually of 7: or 14: years of age.

Presages of Fevers

If many good signs appear at the beginning of a fever, note the signe & degree the moon was in at the decumbiture & the party will recover when the moon comes to the sextile of the place she was then in.[10] Note the place the moon was in at the decumbiture & the view (aspect) the sick body was in when the moon comes to the sextile of that place. If you find ill symptomes of the sick, then you may fear Death, when she [the moon] comes to the quartile of that place. Short maladys are better judged of [than] the long. A good deale of time may produce a great deale of alteration. [Page 12]

6.[11] If Fever happen to women in Child bed, begin the Calculation at the time of her delivery, and take the crisis that way. 7. If the fever continue to the Crisis, which is not often, you may presage bleeding at the nose; it may come on the day of the third Crisis or near it. 8. If the patient bleed at the nose before, he hath an impost[ume] in some of the inferior parts of the body. 9. Flux of blood happens to them under the 30 year, impends to [threatens] them or older. 10. Vehement pain about or near the forehead signifies bleeding at the nose that may save life. 11. Young persons oftener die at the first crisis in fevers than ancient, because their nature is hotter. 12. Old persons oftener die upon relapses because their bodies are weak. 13. Ulcerations in the throat are usually mortal in hot dry cases. 14. Fevers continue longer in ancient people than younger. 15. Ancient people are more subject to quartane agues than young because Saturn causes them.

10. That is, when the moon has gone through one-sixth of its circuit from the time when the patient went to bed.

11. Here Palmer abruptly decides to number (inaccurately) the sentences in this paragraph.

Presages by Squinancys

1. Great pain, difficult breathing; no swelling appear[s] outwardly; usually kills in 4 days.
2. If a squinancy increase on a critical day, break not inwardly nor outwardly, a deadly signe.
3. If a read [red] humour appear outward & fall in again, dangerous.

UVULA

Incision in uvula, Gargarion, or Columella when it is swollen, red, or gross is dangerous; if it be pale or livid, upper part not swollen, it may be open[ed], but purge the body before it [Page 13] if inflamed, blood letting in the arm will serve the turn.

Vomiting in Feavours

A sign when patient seems to sigh. Unless it be not so[12] they will vomit phlegm, choler if they be sick of the stomach.

Of Predominant or hurtful Humours

The Humours are Phlegm, Choller, Melancholy. These humours are more or less in the blood, & out of the blood, either in their proper places, or out of their proper places. In their due places not exceeding (excessive) and of absolute necessity for the good of the body. Choler not exceeding causes expulsion by siege, urine, or otherwise. Melancholy procures appetite, pulse, moderates the heat of choler, keeps the body moist and cold. The Spleen is the seat of melancholy, nourished by it; the Gaule [bladder] the seat of choler and nourished by it; the brains and stomach are furnished with phlegmatical humours.

When Phlegm abounds it causes much spitting, running at the nose, could (cold), swellings, constant f [ever]. When Choler abounds it causeth Vomiting, looseness, intermitting fevers, hot swellings, red pustles (pustules), and other breakings out. When Melancholly

12. Unless they do not sigh.

[abounds], Diseases of the Spleen, hard knotty swellings & meroseness (moroseness).

See the Catalogue of Purging Medicines, Pag. 18 & c. and that will direct for purging the humours. Yet withall note that after purging, sundry other medicines are proper to change the nature of the predominant humour, as a cholerick humour is quenched & altered by cooling things as whey, posset, drink, butter, mild cold herbs if they do not exceed. [Page 14] A Salt humour or Rhum (rheum) is altered, changed by decoctions of Guiacum, etc. Note that these humours are the excremental prt (part) of the superfluities of the first, second or third conconction (concoction). They are encreased & corrupted by unsutable dirt or disorder of the patient, through heat or cold, or by the retention of the accustomed evacuations.

1. The first concoction is in the stomach; if the stomach be cold there is imperfect digestion, much crudities ingendered.

If the Stomach be too hot, causeth much appetite, burnt & chollerick humours, much provocation to vomit, bitter tast in the mouth.

2. [The second] concoction is in the Liver, & meseraical (mesenteric) veins; the excrement of this concoction is Choler. It is sent to the Gaule [bladder] if the Gaul & the passages thereto be not obstructed. Note that the Spleen draweth away the Melancholly juice or excrement and the kidneys, the whey or watery juice or excrement.

3. *As for the last concoction I shall better forbear saying, not willing to dwell any longer upon these matters*, the *difficulty here to be agreed whether there be defect* in 1: 2: or 3: (first, second, or third) concoction: Yet till it be, the way to those medicines *to reach to the 2: 3:* concoction should not be in gross substance & preparations (as most of the ordinary Galenists, both simples & compounds, are.) But [use] such medicines as are free from their passive earth, or passive water, as physitians *put it, write this and take it.* These *are* quintessences, Elixirs, composed of chymical Salts & oyls. This is also called the Balsome Samock (Balsam Samech); without doubt medicines so made exceed all other medicines for the

strengthening of nature to repell the disease, & a few drops at a time, 3 or 4 drops in some *wine* or bear (beer) [blotted], and as some affirm it is an universal [blotted] cleanser, comforter, emptier of all impurities [blotted]: and it may be [Page 15] made of many hearbs or any one hearb by separating the salt and oyl out of any wholsome herb and bringing them into one body, according to art in due length of time.

Balsam Samick (Samech) thus made.[13]

In the first place with a Limbock (alembic) *or better (more) convenient vessel distill them, fret (stir) their water and boil from the herb and do them all.* Then *take the herbs being so distilled and dry them,* calcine *them* & extract out their Salt, then *take this* Salt & mix it with the distilled water and keep *it warm as in the* heat of a Bath for the space of 48 hours or longer; then seperate the *water* either by distilling of it, or Vaporing *it off:* for all the Volatile Salt that is in the distilled water will be mixed with the fixed salt that was made out of the calcined herbs, as may appear by the weight and quantity; then you may add this Salt to more *water* several times as you did at first, then add by Little & little the oyl and in six months it will be brought into a body. Then add Spirit of Wine aromatised; four Drops is a Dose.

The Nature of the 12 Signs of the Zodiack.[14]

Aries is hott & dry, of the nature of fire, good for bleeding.
Taurus, evil for bleeding: dry & cold, of the nature of earth.
Gemini, evil for bleeding, hott & moist, of the Nature of Air.
Cancer, indifferent for bleeding: cold & moist, of the Nature of water.
Leo: evil for bleeding: hot & dry, of the nature of fire.
Virgo: indiffer. for bleeding: cold & dry: of the nature of Earth.

13. The following passage is pure Paracelsian medicine.
14. Each part of the body was governed by a sign of the zodiac. When a day was in that sign, the corresponding member should not be bled.

Libra: is right good for bleeding: hot & moist, of the nature of the air.

Scorpio: indifferent for bleeding: cold & moist, of the Nature of water.

Sagit[tarius] good for bleeding: hot & dry, of the nature of fire.

Capricor[n] cold & dry, of the Nature of the earth. Evil for bleeding.

Aquarius indiff [erent] for bleeding: hot & moist, of the nature of the air.

Pisces indiff [erent] for bleeding: cold & moist, of the nature of water.

Note. Forbear bleeding the member governed of any Sign the day that the Mem[ber] is in it for fear of the great effusion of blood that may happen. Nor likewise when the Sun it in it, for the great danger that may follow thereof. [Page 16]

Phlebotomy or Blood-letting

The Veins in the arm opened are Cephalica *or head vein;* Basilica *or lower vein;* Mediana *or the vein between the two former.*

The mediana is formed of the branches of Cephalica & Basilica, running both in one. Note: *that vein that narrows most is to be bound.* Cephalica *hath neither* Artery nor Sinew near it. The Mediana hath a Sinew just under it. Note that Cephalica sometimes doth not appear, & so sometimes some of the other Veins and sometimes neither of them. In some cases blood-letting saves life, and in some cases destroys it. In abundance of blood & in inflammation of blood, open a vein.

If in the morning about break of day a person useth to sweat, it argues superfluities in the blood. Abundance of blood is known by thickness & troubled consistance of the Urine. Note that where bad and cold blood [blotted], purgation ought to go before. The 2 veins under the tongue are opened for the Squinancy & difficult swallowing. They are both of them apparent ordinarily when the end of the tongue is turned upward. *A woman swelled about the throat but [blot] and cholered, not black but [blot] choler in vein bound give or suffer: for swelling [blot] beside but the throat in squinancy was cured; it [blot] could not [blot] and to [blot] worth drink if parts drain* by cupping *round it [blot] but the neck above the shoulders.*[15] The Veins below the inside of the Ankle are proper in Womenkind to be opened to help *in terms to provoke;* they are small and *do very seldom bleed so freely as the arm.* If you find difficulty in stopping the blood with cotton wool in *the* Head & Arm it [blot] cold [blot] and hand it [blot] the [blot] put in foot. It is counted dangerous to bleed in a dropsy except in the squinancy [blot]. [Page 17]

So it is *in the* Plague *when* any Sore appears or pustule, or fever when any Tumour appears. Yet *it is sometimes good* for bleeding at the nose provided it be at the time of the nose bleeding, to divert the blood another way. *Once I bled D C in the* arm *for the falling sickness hoping it was the cure usually meant; it killed him.* Letting of blood is often profitable for those that have any sore bruises in any part, to divert the humours another way, from flowing to the place bruised, as *they will otherwise be better not to do:* yet withal *it had* need be presently as soon as may be, before the blood be setled, congealed & putrefied. *But wisdom must herein direct as well as otherwise.*

A Coret. (cerote, cerate) *or* Salve for Aches, Strains, for weaknes in *women's* back &c., *be they whites or cholers:*

Rx. a Quart of Sallot Oyl, a pound of Lead, two thirds red & one white. First *take* of Beeswax quarter of a pound, a quart of Oyl & boyl them together & then add the Lead as before & boyle together to a Salve. *Then* add a shilling in Saffron,[16] Nutmeg, Mace & Cloves of each 2 oz. Boyl them in [so as] to mix them a little, & a shilling of oyl of Spike (spikenard). When you add the spice, boyl it in a great Skillet, for any great bruise in head, back or otherwise.

Consumption in the Lungs. For *the* Cough.

Rx. Scabious roots, Elocampane roots, Liquorice, parsley roots, marigold flours [flowers], Maiden hair, Hysop, Sage, Anniseed,

---

15. Much of the shorthand constituting this partly incomprehensible passage was hastily written and is almost illegible. Blotting did not help. Palmer seems to be describing treatment of a woman patient.

16. Enough saffron to cover a shilling.

Horehound, Coltsfoot, Sweet marjoram, figgs, raisens in the Sun, Make a concoction in fair water, F. Syr. S.A. [*Fiat Syrupus secundem Artem*, let a syrup be made according to art]. [Page 18]

Of Working Physick

There be sundry kinds. Some work chiefly by Vomit, some cheifly do work downward, some work both *ways;* some are Violent & dangerous and are not to be used without their proper Correctives added to them. Others are so safe they may be used without their correctives. Some purge Phlegm, some choler, some Melancholy, some most humours & some all humours. To give other medicines then (than) proper purges sutable to the nature of the humour doth often times no good but hurt, especially when the body abounds with ill humours. To imitate nature in these respects is best & *men might learn much this way if their eyes were open. Thus it explains these matters had needs have hard rules to agree (conform to), both having respect to the* age, strength, custom of the patient, season & manner of ordering.

A Vomiting Physick

STRONG KINDS

Stibium or Vitrum Antimonii. Dos[e] 3 or 4 grains to strong grown persons, either the infusion in wine or 2 or 3 grains in (of) the substance in honey. *It is dangerous for* fools or knaves to meddle with it. The purging of it is stopt with the tinc[ture] of wine a spoonfull.

Crocus Metallorum.
Six grains infused all night in 2. spoonfuls of wine is an ordinary dose for ordinary psons [persons] to take, only the wine & lead & the pouder. Or you *may take* 1 oz. of Crocus metallorum in fine powder, 2 oz. or 1½ oz., infuse *it* in a quart of wine for a fortnight's space; twice a day in that time shake *together:* 2 spoonfuls of [Page 19] this wine is an ordinary dose for a man or woman. *It must be to cure one;* you may give more or less according to the age, strength, condition of the party. *If you order them* 6 grans as aforesaid the same may be infused severall times in the same manner. It will work as

well the second time as the first, & if you infuse a quart *when the first quart* [blurred] *one is* [blot] *but may infuse in second or third quart with the same order, and the same dose will do again.*

CAMPBUGE ALIAS CAMBOGE (GAMBOGE) ALIAS GUTTA GAMBA

Dose 6 or 10 or 11 grains in honey or beer or broth. It works safely and surely. I count *it more moderate* then either of the forenamed vomits; it usually works more downwards.

SULPHUR OF ANTIMONY

It is safe, gentle physick, it works most upwards; it is taken in the substance in any drink as bear, Cider, *wine,* broth *or the like.* Dose 7, 8, or 9 grains. Those 4 sorts of vomits work well when rightly ordered.

For Stibium and Campboge see John Woodal.[17] For Crocus Metallorum see London Dispensatory.[18] For Sulphur of Antimony see Schroderus.[19] Crocus Metallorum is stopt with [*i.e.,* its action is stopped by] wine & cloves, stewed together a *little while and now and then give one* a day sometimes I give a little saffron to stop it. These things you may use for Camboge. The Sulphur of Antimony is stopt with a mess of white bread & milk. [Page 20]

SALTS (THAT) PURGE BY COUGH

Use S. John's wort & Polipod.

SALTS THAT PURGE BY URINE

Camomile, wormwood, Gentian, rest Harrow (yarrow?), broom, Bever Cod.

Purge *the* womb in pure yew balm.

Purge by Sweat: Guajacum, Salts [that] ease pain, as of man's blood, stag's blood, goat's blood.

Juice of Elder leaves, 2 spoonfuls in honey & beer, works upwards and downwards. The white juice of wild Flour de luce or stincking

17. *The Surgion's Mate,* pp. 96, 316.
18. 1675 ed., p. 258.
19. *Pharmacopoeia medico-chymica,* 1695 ed., book III, p. 441.

gladen, works freely upward & downward. 2 spoonfulls taken in
bear or broth or whey; it is best of all the Root. *One scruple* is a
Dose.

Powder of Mocoachan (mechoacan) Roots of America, the weight of
6 grains, taken in honey or drink, works freely both ways. It is
stopt with Saffron or Sallot oyl.—yet have a care of medling, I
should sooner use Camboge, Crocus metallorum, Sulphur of
Antimony, than either of those, *though I have had enteric with them
all.*

Groundsel is sometimes used for Vomits; the best way to use it is
two spoonfulls of the syrup at a time. *Some [who] have used it thus
might become sick.*

New England Centaury, a few sprigs of it boyled, works upward &
downward. *Enteric.*

A spoonfull of honey, a spoonfull of fresh butter & a spoonfull of
clear thin Turpentine of the Pine tree is a good Vomit. [Page 21]
But one of the safest things for a Vomit is made of Radish seed,
two spoonfulls. Sod in half a pint of Sack till half be wasted, straine
it, and drink it with 4 spoonfulls of Sallet oyle. By this easy Vomit,
as *some say,* many have been rid of the Cough and much Phlegm
that hath been cloddered. *I like it well; there can be no hurt in it.*

Rx. Cream of Tartar 2 oz. Gallop in fine powder, 2 oz. Sulphur
pulverized, 2 oz., mixed in honey a quartern *but no[t] old.* Dose
as much as a nutmeg in the morning; gives *2 or 3 stools.* [Page 22]

Of Physick working downwards there be a great many sorts, of such
as are moderate & such as are strong.[20]

Syrup of Damask Roses is safe for all sorts of persons.

Syrup of Peach Flowers is safe; they purge stomach and belly chiefly.

Rhubarb of Turk 1 drachm at a time for purging chollerick humours,
for stopping diarrhea, disentery, common flux, bloody flux,
vomiting & loosenes.

Manna 2 oz. at a time for pains inward caused of wind.

Cassia extracted out of the Canes by the Apothecary's art, 2 oz. or
1 oz. at a time, for them [that] are troubled with the stone, stopping

20. Here Palmer begins a discussion of purges.

of Urine, or paines of chollerick humours, or weak persons that cannot use other physick.

Senna is a purger of Melancholly humours. It is commonly used by infusion with Rhubarb & Foods, stewed together all night or some hours boyled in a pott close stopped, and boiled in another Vessel of boyling water. [When] *it has* kept for an hour, strain it out; add a dram of Saffron to it. The Dose of this Medicine: Senna, 1 oz.; Rubarb in powder, one drachm; Seeds, a spoonfull. [Page 23] Order it as above said. Strain it and give a spoonfull of it with a dram of Saffron in it. This prevailes against inward paines as the Chollick works safely, speedily downward, *I* [*obscenity*] *it to extreme.* In the want of Rhubarb of Turk, use Patience root about an ounce or two, thin sliced with the former things, *but it is not so good as the former* [blurred].

An Excellent Purging Medicine

one of the safest & best I ever had the knowledge of; it works only downwards by Stoole. It is called by the name of *The Purging Ale.* It may be given to either young or ould, to women that are not with child and when nature doth not work upon them. It purgeth wind & watry humours & other humours out of all parts that can be & ought to be purged out of the body without any weakening of the body or taking *way* the good colour of [blot] face &c.

Rx. Senna, 3 oz.; Polypody of the oak, 6 oz.; ba (bay) berries huld, 2 oz.; ash Keyes bruised, 4 oz.; Sassafras weed, 2 oz.; Rubarb of Turk, 2 oz. Let these be severally bruised into powder, saving the Senna which must be put in whole. *Let all these* ingredients be putt into a Canvas bag and hang *it* in 3 Gallons of Ale in a barrel that is strong of the second spall as brewers term it. Tye the bag to a hazel [Page 24] stick and let it not touch the barrel by 3 inches nor let it touch the topp. Let it work well about 2 or 3 days before you take it. Drink thereof every morning half a pint, and every evening 3 parts of a half pint. Take some warm broth before dinner, keep warm, & the more you stirr the better *it* will work. It doth not weaken the body nor change the Countenance nor Complexion of you that take it. *It makes the body* lightsome. It will purge no longer than superflous humours do abound. Its for the Dropsy, palsy, Megrim, head ache, pain of the back, stomach, and divers other diseases not here mentioned. It must be taken in either April or September, for the space of a week or a fortnight together.

Another Composition of Senna

Senna, 4 oz.; roots of Monks rhubarb & red madder, of each one half pound; anniseed, rice, of each 2 oz.; scabius & Agrimony, of each a minim. Stew Rhubarb, bruise the seeds & liquorice, breake the herbs with your hands; put them in a close stone pott with 4 Gallons of Strong Ale to steep & infuse the space of 8 dayes. Then drink this liquor for the space of 3 weeks together at the least, for your ordinary drink. And so keep one vessel a preparing while another is a drinking, being always carefull to keep a good diet. It cures [Page 25] Dropsy, yellow Jaundice, all manner of Scabs, breaking out & mangines of the whole body. It purifieth the blood from all corruption, prevails against the green sicknes greatly, and all epilations (depilations) &c.

Note that Senna doth better purge when it is infused or steeped than when it is boyled, for the more it is boyled the less it purgeth, & the more windy it becomes. The easiest way is to steep Senna in Wine so it works with little paine. Because Senna is windy and binds the body after, it is good to mix with things that breake wind, as Cinnamon, Ginger, Annis Seed, fennel seed, raisons of the Sunn, bayberries, &c.

Another

Rx. Senna, 1 oz.; Ginger, half a quarter of an ounce; Cloves, ii; Fennel seed, 2 drams, or instead of it, Cinnamon & Tartar of each, 2 drams. Powder all these. Take 1 dram in white wine before supper. It doth marvelously purge the head.

Another

Rx. Mallows, Elder berrs., Plantain, cruori called sucori, of each a like quantity. *Break* rather a *small* [blurred], Ginger thin sliced, 1 oz.; sassafras roots & Anniseed, of each 1 oz.; Liquorice, 2 oz. Let them be steeped [Page 26] all night in a Pott close stopped set upon the Embers. In the morning let it be boyled with a Pint of Water untill it be half wasted, but let it cease boiling, and put in Senna, 1 oz. Let it steep some hours kept skalding hot. Melt in it Manna, 2 oz. When it is almost cold, take it about 8 times 3 days [blurred], others if it work but little, but if it work freely forbear a day or 2 and so use it a second time or a 3d if you see cause. It may be taken every month in the year in this manner except the 3 hot and 3 cold months. Fair, warm, moderate *weather* is the best weather *to take it*. This is for the Strangury or Voiding of water with paine and difficulty, straining to go to stool, the voiding of blood & slime &c.

Agaric: for the Jaundice, obstructions, to provoke Urine, bringeth down the Mens[es]; against Worms, agues, quotidian & wandring fevers, by drawing & purging gross and cold & phlegmatick humours. The dose is 1 or 2 oz. in powder, mixed with ginger or Sal Gem[mae], or give it in wine wherein Ginger hath been infused. The safest way is to give it with Syrup of Vinigar. *It is for the falling sickness, cureth as but* [blot], inveterate cough, physick, Consumption. It is good for disseases coming of gross, could [cold], and raw humours. Avoid the use of it in any fluxes of the belly. [Page 27]

Turbith

Is to be given as Agarick, in the same Dose, and with the same Concoctors as Ginger. Some hold that the roots of Turbith & Scammoni are the same & that they can find little or no difference.

Coloquintida

The white Pulp taken in the weight of a Scruple opens the Belly mightily, avoids gross phlegm & chollerick humours. It hath the like force if it be boyled or layd to infuse in wine or Ale. The safest use of it is to give the Troches of it called Troches Alhanda. The Dose is 4, 6, to 12 Grains.

Another Receipt of Mr. Arches practice

Rx. Colonquintida *or* apples. Steep a night or two in a quart of wine, and take 4 spoonfulls at a time. When the wine is spent you may steep it in more wine or you may steep half an Apple of Colonquintida in wine. Three of 4: spoonfulls at a time for a night, and take the wine [in] the morning, and the same Coloquintida will do again in wines.

Scammoni

Of it self it is not safe. It may be taken safely mixed with its due Correctours, regarding time, place, quantity & persons that may use it. Diagridium made of Scammoni by art, is taken from 5 grains to 10. or 12. as some affirm; it is safely used in severall sorts of [Page 28] Pills that are compounded of Scammone and other ingredients.

AN ECCELLENT AND SAFE MEDICINE OF SCAMMONI, COMPOUNDED BY JNO. FRENCH & OFTEN PRACTYSED.

Dissolve the Scammoni in the Spir. of wine. Vapour away the one half, then precipitate by adding rose water to it. It will become most white for the black fetid matter will lye on the topp of the precipitated matter, which you must wash away with rose water. Then take that white Gum, being well washed, and dry it: *if you choose you may* powder it & so use it, *for indeed it hath neither smell nor taste*, & purgeth without any offense, and may be given to children or to any that distast physick, in their broth or milk without discerning of it, & indeed it doth purge without any manner of griping. I was wont to make it into pills with oyl [of] Cinnamon, oyl of Cloves which gave it a Gallant smell, and I gave of it *1 scruple* at a time and it wrought moderately, without any manner of griping. But if you please you may take the white gum before spoken of. Dissolve it again in spir. of wine being aromatised with what Spices you please, and this keep to use. This Tincture is so pleasant, so gentle, so noble a purger there is scarce the like in the world, for it purgeth all manner of humours, especially Choler & Melancholly and is very Cordiall. It may be given to those that abhor any medicine, as to children or those of a Nauseous stomach. The Dose is from half a spoonfull to 2: or 3: Note, it must be taken of it self for if it be put into any other [Page 29] Liquor, the Scamoni will precipitate and fall to the bottom.

After this manner you may prepare Jallap, by extracting the Gumme thereof, and then dissolve in Spir. of wines. By this means Jallap will not be so offensive to the stomach as usually it is; for it is the Gum that is purgative and the earthlines that is so nauseous.

Jallap being thus prepared is a most excellent medicine against all Hydronick diseases, for it purgeth watery humours, without any nauseous or griping at all.

Note that if the Gum extracted out of purging or cordial things were extracted, I count them the best of medicines.

Scamoni is black, shining, spungi, brittle, easy broken, light in weight; it shines like Gume, like Glue when its broken in small, not loathsome on tast, not much heating the Tongue; if *it do it is a* sign *it is mixed, part* spurge. These are the signs of good scamoni.

Mirabolans

A fruit comes out of the East Indies like a small lemmon that is of a purging nature. There be 5 kinds, Citrin, Indian, Bollerick (Balearic?), Chebule, Emblic. Some purge Phlegm, Choller, Melancholly. See further of this Woodals first Treatise of Chyrurgions Mate, page 96, and Jno. Gerard, pag. 1317.[21]

Aloes

Aloes as much as a Nutmeg, boyled in a Cup of wine at night, in the first fit of a Fever, cureth it at once as some affirme, & the same Medicine taken twise a year, spring and Fall, prevents a fever, or if it comes it is very small. It usually taken at night in Pills, being made up with honey [Page 30] or wine, or any Syrup sutable. Its very proper to cleanse the stomach, to procure the terms, to cause flowing of the Hemorrhoids, outwardly applyed to them. It stops the flowing of the Hemorrhoids, the bleeding of wounds. It healeth scars & ulcers mixed with proper medicines. Mixed with hogs fatt it dissolveth wens & hard swellings. It is one of the principle ingredients in most of your purging pills.

Of Mechoacans

There be 3 sorts: the 1 is that of Paru: The 2 is Jallap, or black Mochoacan. The 3 sort is wild Mochoacan. I take it to be that of N.

21. *Herball.*

England, yet some through ignorance & boldness [who] use it do not know the exact dose of it, nor the proper correcter of it. The first sort of Mochoacan, the Dose is to a Child 1 scruple to 1½ scruples. To one that is of age & strength, 1 drachm or 2 drachms is not too much. It is not good in hot diseases, for [blurred] or those that are subject to be bound, for it bindeth. Afterwards it purgeth water, phlegm, distillations in the joynts; it provokes Urine, its good for the chollick, pains in the mother. Its said to have all the Virtues that are in Agarick & Rhubarb. Its for the Cough, Catarrh, short breathing, Jaundise, liver, spleen, Kings Evill, skurvie, Gout, inveterate Agues. It purgeth tough and indigested humours in the Stomach & brest. It works most affectually in wine & some say so many peny weight, so many times it worketh.

Jallap

Purgeth phlegm, choller & Melancholly, but cheifly watry humours that more than the former. For the dropsey & green sichness, 1 drachm with wine [Page 31] with Anniseed & Ginger to modify the nausiousnes thereof, whereby it troubles the stomach, and inclines to Vomit. But the best way is to take it with Cream of Tartar, Graines 6. I have had often experiences of the easy manner of its working in this kind & manner. Some have made use of N. England Jallap beaten to powder, steeped in Vinager, and the Vinager two or three times repeated and Vapoured away in the [illegible] untill it be drie. Others have boyled the juice of the root untill it be thick and so dried it to a powder & then taken of peach flours a quart: fill in a glass with water. Let it so stand for a space, straine it out & then add to the water 2 ounces of the aforesaid powder, and use a little of the water for Vomits. But *I have no* experience *but this or the former: so for present I leave it.*

Another Composition of Senna out of James Cook

Rx. Senna, 1½ oz.; Sem Annis & Fennel, of each 2 drams; Agrimoni, Violets, Fumitory, Sabi (sabine?), Strawberries, Mallows, borage, bugloss of each 1 minim; Cremor Tartar (cream of tartar), ½ oz.; Rosemary, ½ minim; clarified whey, 3 quarts. Boyl them till a quart be wasted. Clarify it with whites of Eggs. Let it run through a Cotton bagg of it self. Dose half a pint in the morning, at four in the after noon so much (the same amount). You may encrease or decrease the quantity, as it works to have 3 or 4 stools a day. For dry seat itch after sufficient purging, provoke sweat. [Page 32] [For] Dolor Arthriticus, saith woodall,[22] I seldom use any other purging physick. It purgeth any humours indifferently, it is most in use for running pains of the Gout. Dos. ¹/₂ or 1 dram in some proper syrup.

Of Purging Pills

There be a great many sorts of these in the Dispensatory,[23] and more then needs by farr, yet some of the best I shall insert & of the easiest and safest Compositions.

PILLS TAKEN IN THE MORNING

Pilulae Aureae
Rx. Vide Dispensatory. Dose ½ dram; the utmost dose taken in the morning. Such Pills as have Scamoni alias Diagridium or Colocynthis in them work strongly, and must be taken in the morning, and the body well regulated after then, keeping your chamber and a good fire. Such as have neither Colocynthis nor Diagridium, may best be taken in the evening.

Pill. Cochiae Minor
Rx. Vid. Dispensatory. They purge *water* powerfully. Dose 1 scruple or ½ scruple.

Pill. Rudii
Rx. Vid. Dispensatory. It is one of the dearest yet one of the safest. It cleanseth head, body of Choler, Phlegm & Melancholly. [Page 33] Dose ½ dram: enough for the strongest body. Let the weaker take less, 1 scruple & the weakest less. Keep your chamber; they work very speedily:

22. A reference could not be found in *The Surgion's Mate.*
23. Culpeper's *London Dispensatory.*

PILLS TAKEN AT NIGHT

Pill. Ruffi

Rx. Vid. Dispensatory. 1 scruple taken at night an excellent preservative in pestilential times. They clense the body of humours gott by surfeits. They strengthen the heart and weak stomachs.

Pill. Mastichina

Rx. Vid. Dispensatory. Dose 2 scruples or 1 dram at night. They strengthen the head, & strengthen & cleanse the stomach & work very gently.

Pill. Macri

Rx. Vid. Dispensatory. Good for hurts & bruises, to strengthen the inwarde parts. *Good for stomach and head.* Dose 1 scruple or ¹/₂ dram, going to bed.

Pill. Imperial

Vid. Dispensatory. It cleanseth the body of mixt humours, strengtheneth the stomach exceedingly, as also the bowels, liver & natural spirits. *Good for cold entrails and cheereth the spirits.* Dose 1 scruple or 1 dram at night. It is good to take them many nights together. On the morning drink a draught of warm posset drink & whey. *You may go forth before business. Take them many nights together, for they are proper for such afflictions as can't be carried away at all.* Observe *this* rule in all such Pills are to be taken at night. [Page 34]

Pill. de Hiera cum Agarico

Rx. Vid. Dispensatory. Dose 1 scruple at night. Take them many nights together if you see cause. Its commended for fitts of the Mother, ague, Consumption, disseases of the head, liver, spleen, jaundise, Choller, phlegm, Melancholly humours.

Pilulae de Succino

Rx. Vid. Dispensatory. It preserves the stomach from all Diseases, suffers nothing to purify therein, expells all humidity from the Stomach, cleanseth the same. They that use it often have never any more paine in the Stomach. It causes mirth, strengthens the heart & head, cleanseth Reins & womb exceedingly. It amends the evill state of a Womans body, strengthens Conceptions & takes away what hinders it. It greatly purgeth choller & phlegm & leaves behind a binding, strengthening quality behind it. Pills of Amber purge the Head and Womb.

As for more Sorts of Pills and working physick Vid. Dispensatory. [Page 35]

General Rules to be observed, by them that take physick

The Physick which you take in the morning that is purging or vomiting.

1. If it can be, let it be betimes in fair weather. If not fair, yet let the Season be warm. Keep warm, keep house. The longer the Stomach is empty before you take it, the more apt it is to digest, & less apt to work.
2. What drink or broth you take, let it be warm & often.
3. Be sure to keep awake, & Stirr, the more you stir the better it works.
4. If it work much, keep as still as you can, and keep the bed.
5. If it do not stop in short time, use means to stop it.
6. An hour after it hath done working, you may either sleep, or Eat. Let it be something of easy disposition.[24]
7. If it work much upwards, use means to turn it down. If you are weak, a Clyster or Suppository some times will do it. Sometimes Oximel of Squill or wine with Cloves stewed in it, or brandy, or Rum.
8. Have a care of Cold in the time of working or after or before. Some kind of physick after taking cold will continue working till blood come.
9. After physick some cleansing, altering hot drink is good to prevent extreme costiveness. [Page 36]
10. Be sure to give moderate physick to weak body's & stronger to strong body's.

24. Easily digested.

11. Be sure to use corrective & such physick as stand in need of Correcters.
12. If your physick work but little & the distemper ould & have long afflicted the body, it is not one potion but several must be made use of, for disseases will not at once have moved out of the body, & one potion doth but fit the body for another.
13. Let Women have a care of taking Vomits when they lye in Childbed, their terms are at that time stopt, or at other times when they are upon them, or evident tokens of them.
14. Have a Care of working physick when the body is very much wasted with lingring or long sickness, or losse of much blood.

Of Extream Costiveness

Those that have been much afflicted with extream costiveness & inward paines, I have used several things to good advantage, yet those things which have helped at one time would not at another. Sometimes I have used to profit Clysters of the decoction of wild flag roots with blue flowers. Stamp the roots and boyl them, & strain them out & so give it. Sometimes this has failed, and clysters of childs uren hath done. Sometimes a [Page 37] suppository of honey & Aloes helped when other things failed. Sometimes a potion of [blot] 2 ounces of manna, hath helped when other things failed. Sometimes Pill. Ruffi have done good in this case & anoynting the Belly with an Oyntment of Wormwood, Rew (rue), Sage seeds, Camomile, peneroyal, made with fresh butter. Smoak of Tobacco blown up the boddy[25] I have known to give present ease. And Sometimes using Ungt. Nicotiana. Some had anoynting with ol chym. absinth 8. or 4, or 6 drops. Once with giving of clysters of flour deluce roots, stampt & boyled anonyting with the former Compound oyntment & giving of Aloes in pills, all this being used together, brought to such a looseness. They were stopt with a decoction of red oak bark in drink.

---

25. An enema of tobacco smoke.

These Medicines are Commended

Rx. Aloes, Bulls gaule, Sal Gem, oyl. /F. unguent. Anoynt the fundament; provokes to stools presently. Let it be within the fundament. Or Rx. Bulls gaule bound to the Navel with tow. Or Rx. Coloquintida (colocynthis) mixed with honey, bulls gaule; make a pill. One pill taken moves the belly presently. Vid: Vade Mecum, the broad paper book with wash leather cover.[26] [Page 38]

Of Extream Looseness or Fluxes

If it comes with a Vomit, give working physick in the beginning while they can bear it, or at least give some gentle thing to turn it downward, as Syr. of damask roses, or Manna, Aloes or Rhubarb.

If it be only Vomiting, give a Vomit of Sulphur of Antimony. I have found it profitable. If both way is working, I have found rose syrup do good. It turns the Course downward. If it be only downward, give gentle purging physick. This is the best thing while there is strength.

Some Commend these things

1 dram of album graecum in powder. Rosted Cheese in powder given, seed of Coriander drunk, powder of ox maw given in drink. A Certain physitian cured divers patients with this only medicine.

A Certaine Child had a looseness for several dayes, sometimes vomiting. [The child was] about a year and quarter ould. After the use of several things this proved the most effectual medicine, viz. Rx. white oak bark boyled in water with Cloves & mace & seeds, a Crust of wheat bread. By gods blessing the looseness quickly eased.

Another Child a year old had a looseness & vomiting after divers medicines. I gave it a Vomit of the infusion of Crocus Metall. It vomited twice & that day the Vomiting ceased & the looseness mitigated: *It will blast* [line blotted]. [Page 39]

An Indian Woman Vomited so much that she vomited blood. She was presently cured by giving her 3 times going over after another

---

26. This suggests that the present vade medum was derived from an earlier draft.

decoction of spere mint. A certain boy followed with a flux in winter time. He could not keep his bed, which continued for many nights. Was cured by taking 4 gutt. of chym (chymical) oyl of Peneroyal, in a little sugar, going to bed. *He took it with bark. It cured him: Since this, Master Fuller, I have done good to several* others with the same oyl.

Of Chymical Oyls

Oyl of Hysop, a drop to anoynt the temples in great paine of the head as in fevers, agues & it is an excellent thing, I know by experience. It is also good for shortness of breathing, for the Cough to procure sweat, and to procure Womens sickness. Taken some time together it hath done good in this respect when other things have failed.

Oyl of Peneroyal

For coldnes of the stomach, for inward paines, for [blotted], for the green sicknes, for procuring of Sweat, for could diseases of the inward parts.

Oyl of Mint

For Wormes in children, for Vomiting, and loosenes, inward paines of could cause. [Page 40]

Oyl of Wormwood

For stomach paines, to clense the stomach and Veins of phlegm & choller. Outwardly used to scatter swellings that have not been of long Continuance. To anoynt the Stomach or belly or sides or other parts pained, but a few drops will serve the turn at a time. Drop 2 drops into the Navill for the Chollic & paines in the bowells. Anoynt the swelling of Wounds. For Costiveness take 3 or 4 drops at a time at night going to bed. It may be given in almost any disease, as a Cordial, when other hot oyls cannot well be taken, yet where blood is lost out of the body, by nose, wounds, or otherwise forbear (do not give) it. Taking it inwardly, yet outwardly after the blood is stopt, it is a very good balsam.

Of Oyl of Anniseed

For Cough, short breathing, inward paines, or most diseases or obstructions or stopage in the inward parts.

Oyl of Cummin Seed

For all disseases of wind, paines in any part of the body. Oyl of Fennel Seed of the same nature. [Page 41]

Oyle of Spices

OYL OF CINNAMON

For Cold disseases such as are speechles. It is as good as Natural Balm for wounds & ulcers, prevails against diseases coming of cold, helpeth Women in Travail.

OYL OF CLOVES

Stayeth ye putrifcation of the bones in old and new ulcers, asuages the paine in the teeth from a Cold Cause. It heals wounds, diseasses, wind, digesteth cold humours. Causes a sweet breath. *The Oyle of Mace* hath the same virtues as the oyle of Cloves.

OYLE OF NUTMEG

Of use for cold diseases of the Head, for Strengthening of the Memory for the obstructions of all the inward diseases coming of cold.

Oyl of Peter

Some of the ancient writers do affirm that it comes out of rocks, as in Italy & other parts in the world. It is profitable for the palsy, giddines of the head, for the falling sicknes. This oyl is principally used outwardly, very profitable used outwardly for setled paines in any part of the body. A certain man with a few drops of this oyl was cured of a pain in his huckle bone that disenabled labour. Another man was cured with once using of it of a paine in his huckle bone that was tedius to him to stirr. Another man with a paine and swelling in his back had help by the use of this oyl. It is excellent good in bruises & it is affirmed that this oyl doth penetrate & digest all excremental matter.[27] [Page 42]

Oyl of Eggs

This oyl is made of the yolks of Eggs. It cures burnings & scaldings without any fever, excoriations, chaps, sore eyes, cutts, takes away sweating coming of hott causes in the begining.

Oyl of Vitriol

Is exceeding sharp & cold. The mixing of this oyl with syrups, conserves, decoctions, or waters makes such things cold as it is mixed with all. It makes them tart or sowereth (soureth) & is profitable so given in fevers pestilential, falling sicknes, palsy, stopping of urine & most *other diseases*, but observe to drop so many drops into any liquid matter as will make it tast a little sower & always when it is used shake it up from the bottom.

Oyl of Sulphur

This oyl is distilled from Brimstone and is used a few drops for hot disseases in water or beer, for fever, for the falling sickness, shortnes of breathing, & diseases of the lungs.

The outward use of these two last oyls is to cleanse ould scars & ulcers, to take away the Callous flesh, which must be done very warily in this wise following.[28] Take a knitting needle or a bodkin or probe or such like instrument & twist a little cotton wool about it, & just dip it into the oyl, & lightly touch the callous flesh, & this must be done sundry times, as you see cause requires, for wounds or ulcers cannot be healed, till this callous flesh be taken away. [Page 43]

Oyl of Turpentine

Cures wounds both inward & outward, & cures aches of the Limbs, is often times one of the special ingredients in several sorts of balsams.

---

27. An example of the widely held belief that many externally applied remedies could cure internal diseases. "Rock oil" later became a well-known patent medicine.
28. Note the use of sulphuric acid as a caustic.

OBSERVATION

The Oils of Herbs and Spices are commonly mixt with Sugar or Conserves or other sollid medicine, but for them that cannot so take them, mix a few drops first with sugar & then disolve that sugar in wine or bear & the oil will not be so apt to swim on top, *for if it swim on top it can't so well be taken.*

Oil of Amber

Is taken often for the palsy, for Women in Travail, & counted profitable in most diseases as a Cordial.

Oil of Sage & Rosmary

Are counted very excellent in diseases of the Head, as the palsy, apoplexy, &c.

OBSERVATION

These kind of Chymical Oils though they are hot in tast & strong in smell, yet to those that can & will take them they are the best of medicines. [Page 44]

Oils not chymical, made by infusion or digestion or Concoction are these. Oil of Camomile, oil of Roses, or Wormwood, or oyl of Elder-flours, or oyl of water Lilly flours, and any of them good for pains and swellings that have not been of long continuance. But if paines & swellings are removed by them, then purge the body presently except some just cause to hinder, as some sickness, great weakness, or unsutable season of the year. Otherwise such remedys prove worse than the disease most commonly. Pulvis Arthriticus is used with success for all sorts of gouty pains, yet in the want of it other things may be used to purge such humours, as Jallap or other things that work safely downwards, for this is an ordinary Rule that there is no Medicine so good but some thing else may be as good.

These forsaid oils & many others may be made with sallot oil, fresh butter, Cream, hogs fat, or any other oil, the Herbs being steeped in it.

Ointments are Commonly made in the same manner as the foresaid oil, but they are made of many things mixt together & some times with wax added & then they are called Cerets (cerates) &

some of their thin ointments that are put into Soars are called Liniments, yet Liniments, Cerets & unguents do but little differ, as a great Tree and a shrub. [Page 45]

Unguents of the Apothecary shop that follow are the best & safest.

Unguentum Aegyptiacum

Vid. Dispensatory. For burning & scalding, to take hot swellings away & inflammation in wounds that hinder the healing.

Linimentum Gummi Elemi

Vid. Dispens. It eases pains in Soars, heals ulcers but is cheifly used for Wounds & Ulcers in the Head.

Basilicon

Vid. Dispens. It aswages pain, digests, procurs matter, cleanses soars, incarns, and heals.

Unguent. e Nicotiana

Vid. Dispens. for the Composit [ion] & Vertues.

Unguentum Apostolorum

Vid. Dispens. It consumes Corrupt & dead flesh, makes flesh soft which is how it cleanseth wounds, ulcers & Fistulas & restores flesh when it is wanting.

If you would be acquainted with any more see the Dispensatory. By the same Rules may ointments be made either of Herbs or flours either hot or could, simple or compound, according to the discretion of them that practice.

Vid. Pag. 52: Anodine oyntment. [Page 46]

Of Plasters

Emplastrum Cymino

Vid. Dispensatory. This is good for windy ruptures & to dispell wind. It asuageth swellings, taketh away old aches coming of bruises.

An excellent remedy for the wind chollick. Often proved & always
of good success, by Culpeper.

Diachilon

There be 3 sorts, vid. Dispens. and they are used to soften swellings but the best sort is called Diachilon mag. cum gummi.

[Emplastrum] Oxycroceum

Vid. Dispens. It Comforts the Limbs, is good for [blotted] &
diseases, cold humours. It is used for straines and bruises, paines,
to Limbs broken or out of joynt, & is sometimes used for the said
things being mixed with Paracelsus plaster.

Emplastrum Sticticum Paracelsi

Vid. D. This is commonly used by most chyrurg[eons] for Sores,
Swellings & Ulcers, both young & old.

Emplastrum de Meliloto

Of it there be 2 sorts, both Simple and Compound. It is commonly
used to break swellings, & to heale them & also it healeth other
Soares. [Page 47]

Emplastr. ad Herniam

Vid. Disp. It is used for Ruptures, strengthens the back, stops
fluxes & prevents miscarriage.

Empl. Hystericum. Vid. pag. 166

It is good for Hysterical fitts, being applyed to the Navel. Being
laid to a Womans navil, a hole cut in the plaster for the navil to work,
it cures the fits of the mother.

Diapalma alias Diacalcytheos

Vid. Disp. It is a very drying plaster, profitable in green wounds
to brak & prevent putrif.

Flos Unguentorum. Vid. Dispens.

It dissolves & digests humours. It is drawing, cleansing & good for strains. It will draw out thorns stuck in the flesh & is good applyed to any pain, as of the Reynes (reins) Spleen, or liver &c. See the dispens. for more Sorts. An Artist may make plasters as he sees cause, by boyling stampt herbs, or flours, in oyl, butter, or hogs fatt & then strain out the herbs & add to the fatt or oyl, rosin, turpentine, pitch, having issue to bring it to a body,[29] these kind of plasters so made will do as well, yea & farr better then many of those that come from beyond seas, for that which is farthest fetch'd & dearest bought, is not alwayes the best, except it be for them that have great purses.[30] [Page 48]

Emplastrum Nigrum called the Black Plaster

Rx. White Lead, 1 lb., black lead, red lead, of each 1 lb., Sallet oyl, a quart; bees wax, 1/2 lb.; Venice turpentine, 2 oz. Boyl these together to a plaster. The longer you boyl it the blacker it will be. This is a good plaster for sores old or new that are inflamed but in cold weeping sores other plasters are better.

Emplastrum Epispasticum

Rx. Mustard seed, Euphorbium, long peper, of each 1 1/2 dram; stavesacre pelletory (pellitory) of Spain of each 2 drams; [gum] ammoniacum, Bdellium, Sagapen, of each 3 drams; Cantharides in powder, 1 dram; ship pitch, Rosin, yellow wax, of each 1 1/2 drams; Turpentine, as much as is sufficient. This is good to draw blisters in the neck for the tooth ach, or for Rhume in the Eyes &c. Some draw (raise) blisters in this manner following: Take a small spoonfull of kie (kye) meal, mix it with a little vinagar into past, spread it upon a cloth, and sprinkle the pouder of half a dozen cantharides thereon.

Also Rosa Solis will draw blisters, as also May Weed alias Pis-a-bed,[31] the flowers stampt & wett with Vinegar, Sanicle leaves & so

29. That is, to cause a discharging sore to come to a head.
30. An important rationalization for the colonial physician.
31. Mayweed was regarded as a diuretic. Hence this remedy was also thought capable of draining a blister.

will Crowfoot root stamped & aplyed. Each of those forementioned will draw Blisters. Probatus est. [Page 49]

Cordial Medicines & Sweating

These Medicines are of sundry Sorts & forms. Some are liquid & some are sollid. The End and use of these Medicines, are to Comfort the Spirits & defend the heart & they are used to such persons as cannot safely take working physick and sometimes they are taken after working physick. Observe by the way that ordinarily diseases begin in the Stomach[32] & in the beginning may be easily expelled either by Vomit or Siege, but such is the Misery often times that before any means can be used, partly by the neglect of those whom it doth concern, & other causes, yet the patient is not capable of taking working physick. For in this time much of the disease is sucked into the Veins & then sweating Medicines is to be applyed, as Treacle water, Spirit of Saffron, Bezoar water, Aqua Celestis, or in want of these great Cordials, Mithridate, Diascordium, Venice Treacle, London Treacle, Diatessaron, besides chymical Elixirs, Chymical Oyls, Antimonium Diaphoreticum, rightly made. James Cook highly extolleth a preparation of hearts horn, & saith that it provoketh sweat more than bezoar & is thus prepared. First of all Take Elder flowers & steep them in white wine Vinegar & change the Vinegar with fresh flowers several times, letting them always stand in the Sun in hot weather. This being thus prepared, then take harts horn burnt white & heat very hott & squench (quench) 6 or 7 times in this Vinagar of Elder flowrs & then dry it. The Dose is 20 gr. mixed with any other medicines.

Observe by the way, that in such diseases where many die & in short time whether it be the plague [Page 50] or small pox, or any pestilential fevers. It is counted a sure Rule by some to shune working physick, & apply to Cordials, but certainly they do little good, if they do not procure sweat plentifully, but there is great hazard of

32. Hence such diseases were due to failure of the first concoction and to formation of the resulting "crudities," or undigested substances.

taking of cold. It will be very dangerous to the patient whether it be hot or cold.

As for directions about sweating see more hereafter. The Dose of these medicines must be according to the age & strength & condition of the patient. The Dose of Mithridates is the quantity of the small Nutmeg.[33] London treacle, such a quantity. Venice Treacle, the quantity of an Indian bean. Diatessaron, the quantity of a small nutmeg. These may be taken on the point of a Knife or they may be dissolved in the water of Carduus distilled or Rue or Angelica, or dragons [blood], or in any of their decoctions.

Mr. Chancy's great Cordial drink

for the Plague, small Pox, or other pestilential Diseases. Also it is good for Surfeit, the Meazels &c.

Rx. Rue, Sage, of each 1 minim; boyl them in spirits of Malmsy or Muscadine or Sack, untill a pint be wasted. Strain it. Set it over the fire again & add it to a peny worth of long peper of Ginger, 1 oz.; Nutmeg, 1/4 oz.: beat them and [Page 51] let them boil a little. Add to it 6 peny worth of Mithridate, as much London Treacle. Add to it good aqua Vitae, & strong Angelica water, a quarter of a pint. Take it warm a spoon or 2 morning & evening, & sweat should pour. If it come freely do not force it. This alone will help by god's blessing. John French speaks of the same & highly commends it & leaves out the aqua Vitae.

Amongst Cordials may be ranked Syrups, Juleps, Conserves & preserves. Syrups & Juleps are made of decoctions or distilled waters of herbs or flours. Some of the best are Syr. of Horehound, Scabius, Angelica, Roses but the Syrup of wild Roses are counted the most cordial, to cause sweat, & seige. Next for to purge gently are syr. of Damask Roses.

Take as many Roses as water, boyl them a great while in a pot close stopped & set in water, then strain it out & adde so much sugar that is white as will make it into a Syr.

---

33. A mass equal in size to that of a small nutmeg.

Conserve of Marigold for trembling of the Heart

Conserve of Red Roses to coole & stop fluxes

Conserves are made of Herbs or flowers either raw or boyled, made with fire or without. You must to 1 oz. of herbs of flowers adde 3 oz. of sugar stamped together. If you make them by boyling adde a little water to them, & so stew them being stirred [Page 52] with Sugar in water till they are soft & the water boiled away.

Conserve of Calamint flowers, a great Cordial to move sweat, to defend the heart & proper for the Green Sicknes.

Conserves of Rue are of the same Natures. So is preserved Angelica Roots. And Fruits are preserved with Decoctions in & with Sugar.

Pulvis Bezoarticus Anglicus 2 drams given in the water of sweet Chervil moves Sweat plentifully.

An Emulsion of Poppy seed, Millet, Carduus Benedictus &c. good after sweating in Feavers.

Anodine Oyntment

Take rose leaves & rott them in may butter a long time, then boyl it up with Camomile.

Another ungt. to ease paine, take away and scatter swellings, good for burnings. Rx. Rose leaves. Rott them in butter, then take Johnswort flowers, Clovenswort, Camomile &c. F. ungt. [Page 53] Some Collections out of James Cook concerning Chyrurgery here inserted.[34]

Corruption of Bones[35]

They are black, feel rugged. Flesh Spungy, of a livid colour. Tents reaching to the bone. Smell. Quitter flow too plentifully, or thin & shrinking. If it skin (heal over) & breake out again, if it be long in healing, rebell against proper Medicine.

Bare the bone by incision, Caustick, or dilation. Scale the bone cum Pulv. Euphorb. If deep, by actual Cautery scale the bone, or use the tincture of Mars, in this book described, Page 233.

34. James Cooke was the author of *Melleficium chirurgiae* and *Supplementum chirurgiae*.
35. Osteomyelitis.

Note that the Salts of Herbs are good to cleanse ulcerated Soars, being put in dry. Of Flesh discoloured there is 4 sorts. Red, Yellow, Livid, or black. Red proceeds from heat, or by blood offending in quality or quantity. If the body be plethorick, or too hot & fervid, for the first bleed & Scarrify the part & apply Leeches. If it happen through defect of the Hemorroids or Menstr. (menstruation), procure their fluxion 1. by applying of Leeches. 2. By using Elixir proprietatis or Pil. Pestilential, being taken sundry times. [Page 54] For the Second open Saphene (saphenous vein) in the foot, use sutable diet.

Livid flesh [is caused] by corrupt & black blood setled in the part. For this you are to scarrify, apply leeches after foment (fomentation) with oximel dissolved in aqua Card. benedicta. If it proceed from cold that is perceived by the temper of the part apply this: Rx. a Turnip & a Radish Root. Scrape these two and add to them of the pouder of Mustard seed, 1 oz.; Caryophil. pulv., 3 drams; Oyl Linceed & Jugland, q.S.F. Catapl [asm]. Apply this warm. It hath cured several Gangreens.

Black [flesh] which may either proceed from heat or could. If from heat, an inflammation went before it. If from cold, lividity did preceed. That is a sign of mortification, especially if no heat or feeling did remain. In both these cases the parts are to be scarrified profoundly, using a Lixiv [ium]. wherein is decocted wormwood containing Scordium, Card. Bened., flours of Camomile, Dill, Melilot; after, fill the incision of the Scarification with some of the medicament following, using a fether.

Rx. Farin. fab. hord. & ereb. (farina fabarum, hordeorum, et erebinthi), of each 4 oz., Lixivium Mitioris, 4 lbs. Boyl to a cataplasm. Then adde oximel, 2 drams; unguent. Egyptiae, 1 oz. Mix all well. Continue the use of these Medic [ines] [Page 55] till the part returns to the Natural Colour.

Of Swellings

These are hot or cold, new or old. Could swellings are hard & difficult to breake. They usually are long, low, white, and pale, lesse painful then hot swellings. Hott swellings are much sooner broken.

They bunch up round, & are red & high coloured. For the beginning the best way is to take often purging physick, or as the strength & Condition of the party will bear.

Note that usually your swellings of long continuance do foule corrupt the bone. These old swellings being broke and running are usually called Ulcers. When the bone is foule, the Soar cannot be healed without these Rules following.

1. Divert the humours away from the place, if it may be, by working physick.
2. Comfort & strengthen & warm the part, or take away unnatural heat if there be need.
3. Scale the bone if foule by sutable medicines, as [unguentum] Egyptiacum, Apostolorum, or the Tincture of Mars, for it is the best.
4. Remove by Causticks, Cauterys or dissolvers the hard & callous flesh. Note that your fixed salts of vegitables, a small quantity put into an old or ulcerate soar, doth cleanse it to admiration & procure good quitter. It must be used now & then. Though it be very painful it makes sweet a [Page 56] stinking soar & is far more safe then Arsenick or precipitate & can do no hurt though others may. It hath cured very foule soars, using no other Medicin.[36]

Lucatellus (Lucatello's) Balsam

Vid. Dispens. This is for wounds, bleeding, scalding, bruises, Strikes (strokes), Sciatica, choll [er]. 2 drams given in white wine. For Worms given every morning, Sinews shrinking.[37] It ripens all Apostumes, healeth them, cureth Cancers & ulcers, aches, cold humours, palsy & appoplexy, could disseases of the braine. Good for head ach, Temples, Nostrils being anointed. [Good] against poison & surfeits, being taken in Sack, for the plague, Fistuloes, small Pox, Meazels. Draweth away broken bones, or any putrification, easeth paine, hinders inflamation in Wounds.

36. Now Palmer has ended his notes from Cooke and returns to a list of remedies.
37. Meaning uncertain. Perhaps this refers to stiffness of the joints.

OF PHYSICK AND CHYRURGERY

Another Balsam; its said to heale a Wound in 24 hours.

Rx. ol. Hyper [ici], Lumbricorum, terebinth, Mastic ana 1 oz.
Misce & apply it hott with Lints. [Page 57]

Another Sort of Balsam

Rx. Johns wort, Clowns wort, Yarrow, Sollomons Seale, Mullen,
plantain, Knot-grass, wild Tansy, Comfry. Stamp the Herbs to mash
with fresh hogs fatt in a Morter. So let them stand 2 or 3 days, then
boil them. In the boyling ad a little turpent [ine]. Let them stand 2
or 3 dayes more, then boil them & straine them. This for wounds,
bruises, hot swellings, for burnings & scaldings.

Note that your oyl of Turpentine of the Apothecary is a good
Balsam of it self for new wounds. So is Unguent Nicotianae.

Balsam of Hypericon

Rx. Leaves , flowers & seeds of Saint Johns wort, Stampt & put
in a glass with Olive oyl & set in the Sun for sundry weeks. Strain
it out, & adde more of the same to the said oyl & set it in the sun
as before. This is of the Colour of Blood, a precious remedy for deep
wounds, & those that go through the body, for Sinews prickt or any
wound made with a Venomed weapon.

Another

Rx. White wine, 2 pints; oyl Olive, 4 lb.; ol. Terebinth, 2 lb.;
Leaves flowers seeds of Hypericon, two great handfulls, gently
bruised. Put them altogether in a double glasse & set it in the sun
8 or 10 dayes. Then boyl them in the same glasse in Balnea Maria,
i.e., in a Kettle of water with straw in the bottom, wherein the glasse
must stand to boyle. [Page 58]

If you dare venture it, its best to boyl them in a stone, or bottle
of Pewter. Straine the liquor from the herbs, & do as you did before
in adding like quantity of herbs, flowers and seeds, not any more
wine, so have you a great secret. John Gerard saith, I knowe there
is not in the world a better balsam, no, not natural Balsam itself, for
I dare undertake to cure any such wound, as absolutely in each
respect if not sooner & better as any man whatsoever shall or may

with natural Balsam. John Gerard so, page 433 D.[38] Se what Gerard writes of Theremac (Theriac), Adders tongue. See what he speaks of Tobacco, page 288 A. [Page 59]

Flux of blood at the Nose

Some one was cured by taking a purge. When it wrought, the flux stopt when many former means failed.

Some have stopt it with an Actual Cautery to the Soals of the feet of each foot. *Riverius* saith that 1 dram of Spice Nardi in broth or plantain water or other fitt (suitable) liquor the most present remedy.

Gout Pains

Bath with wollen stuffs diped in water of frogg as hot as may be. Dip a cloth about the place, another a top of it & so go to bed after bathing a good while first. If need be, dresse it so again the next day.

The Frogge Water thus made

Rx. Frogg spawn, fill an earthen pott there with, cover it & sett it in the ground, half a foot deeper than the pott is high, being covered with Earth. Let it stand so two or 3 weeks. In the same time it is turned into water strain it & keep it in Bottles, for use as a-foresaid. Oyl of frogge is good for the same malady. In the use of the water, one in Lichestshier (Leicestershire) gott a good estate thereby.[39] If need be, dresse the next morning with the water in the same manner.

Observation that if the gout invade with a Fever, hot sweating medicines are not to be administered except such as be temperate, as this which is excellent. Corn[u] cervini usti, 1 or 2 scruples. See of this in the discourse of Cordial medicines before.

---

38. *Herball*, p. 433D.
39. An unusual reward from a grateful patient.

Iliaca Passio

Some Commend Cremor Tart. (cream of tartar) a liberal dose, also Cow dung new made & gathered. Apply 3 times a day. A pound of Caule of a Ram, dissolved & taken inwardly.

Of Wens

Some have been cured with a plate of Lead besmeared with Quicksilver, though they could [Page 60] not be broken.

Riverius in his observations cured 3 with sorrel leaves roasted under the Embers, & applyed for many days. They may be tyed about the Roots till they fall off themselves.

Diet Drink for wounds by Gun-shot or otherwise. Drives out Iron, wood, Lead, and all other extranious bodys. It heals more in a week than all other medicines without it in a month.

Rx. Allchymilla,[40] bet[a] rub[ra], pirole Sannicul., Vinc. pervinc., Virga aurea, Sem. Angelic., of each equal parts. Let the herbs be shred small, Seeds powdered, mix this powder with the herbs.

Take of this, 1½ oz.; renish wine, 2 lbs. Boyl them in a close vessel. Make a clear decoction. The dose is two or 3 spoonfuls, 3 times a day, this when the paine & inflammation is past and the wound comes to digestion. See in Gerard or some other Herbal the Latine Names of these Herbs, to know what they are called in English. [Page 61]

Aches or paine in the Limbs. Jelly of Harts horn, made with scrapings of harts horn, strong Ale & Mutton fatt, any sort of strong waters, with Ox Gaul & Oyl of Camomile in an Oyntment.

Ach in any part [41]

Rx. Pigeons dung, 4 oz.; strong ale, sheep suet, Camomile. Stew them together. F. Catapl. & apply it on a cloth all night.

---

40. An abbreviation for *Achillea millefolium*, q.v.
41. Here the author begins an alphabetical consideration of ailments.

Now if the body be strong, Vomits, purges, letting blood, sweatings, the use of Cupping glasses are all useful.

Observations

If the place pained be colder then other parts, anoint often with your chymical oyles, to keep & defend from cold & bring the place to its natural temper. Oyl of Mint, Peneroyal, Wormwood, Calamint, Isop [hyssop], time [thyme], oyl of peneroyal, any of these used a few drops at a time, for several times.

For setled pains in a Limb, oyl of Peter excelleth. For running pains, Issues are good, made several ways.

Agues & Fevers

In the beginning Vomits, blood letting usually help in strong bodys. In weake bodys before the fitt come, use Carduus posset, with Mithridate, or Treacle a little before the fitt come & sweat thereupon. Or Treacle water, 3 spoonfulls; Syrup of Saffron, one; mix together & give it & sweat after it. Or Antimony Diaphoret rightly prepared, a few graines, 6 or 8 or 10, or 3 or 4, as the patient is, or distilled water or wormwood, or salt of wormwood, Carduus in wine, or Saffron in wine &c. In the beginning of most distempers that may [Page 62] be done quickly with Gods help, yet afterwards cannot be done for many pounds, when at first 3, or 4, or 5 shillings may be sufficient before nature be weak.

Note that some Fevers are mortal, as putrid fevers, spotted fevers. If sweating Medicine be used, for they are most cheif [preferred], the greatest difficulty is for fear of taking cold in the time or a short time after, for it often proves very destructive to divers [patients], as lamentable experience hath proved. And to Women that enjoy not their Lunary Tribute [menses] & to children that do abound with worms.

To the former, to take away the cause when very weake is a difficult task & harder then many are aware of. Therefore being forewarned, be forearmed in time. And [remember] to trust to cool-

ing Medicines in fevers. The Neglect of Diaphoretic Cordials is as
thin [inadequate] as to rely on the Reed of Egypt.

Almons of the Throat inflamed

This Malady hinders Speech, swallowing and breathing, must
needs be grievious & dangerous. It is known by the rednes & swelling of the parts, about the throat. The cure is by purging downwards
& bleeding & applying of cupping glasses to the shoulders & neck,
by pricking the inflamed parts of the throat by a Lancet tyed to a
flat stick, by bleeding under the tongue, in one of the Veins or both,
houlding warm water in the mouth, while the patient bleedeth. Astringent Gargarisms are profitable made with honey, spring water,
Allom (alum), Clysters that work strongly & cooling drinks to coole
the heat of the [Page 63] inward parts, to sit up much & ly down
but little, to sleep sitting in a chair upright.

Annurisme (Aneurysm) and the Cure

It is a soft humour made by the pricking of an Artery, most commonly in blood letting, also by the opening of Artery's unskillfully
performed & negligent cured. Some times they happen in the Throats
of women after painful travil. It is a soft humour, yeilding to the
impression of the fingers.

The cure is by applying of cloths double steeped in nightshade
juice or house leek with one oz wheyey cheese mixed therewith, or
Unguent de Bolo, or Emplastr. contra rupturam, or a thin plate of
Lead applyed.

That which comes by Blood-letting may be holpen (helped) by
applying the pouder of Aloes with the hairs of a hair (hare) skin. It
had need be done as soon as the Artery is pricked. Let the young
Chyrurgeon take heed he do not rashly open any artery Annurisme,
except small & in some ignoble part. Let it be done on this manner.
Cut the skin that lys over it untill the Artery appears, then seperate
it with your knife from the particles about it. Then thrust a blunt
crooked needle with a thred in it under it [the artery], bind it & then

cut off the thread, & so expect the falling off the thread, while nature covers the orifice of the Artery with new flesh.[42] The rest of the cure will soon be cured, as simple to.

Back and weaknes thereof

Pills of Turpentine made up, with Cinnamon & Nutmeg in powder. Take 3 or 4 at a time, for several nights together. This is good for running of the Raynes. [Page 64]
A good quantity of Ox Pizel boyled in Muscadine till it be thick, strain it, & take 4 or 5 spoonfulls at a time, for 4 or 5 dayes together.[43] Also a Tansy made of clary & nutmegs and Eggs often eaten.

Back, heat thereof

Rx. Ungt. Fridg. Galeni, Housleek Juice, 1 oz.; Mirtle, 3 drams; Camphor, 1 dram. Make these into an oyntment in a leaden Mortar and let the back be anointed therewith. Some times the ungt. fridg. Gall. is sufficient.

To cleanse the Back and purge the Kidneys

Parsly Roots and Pellitory of the Wall boyled together in ale. Take it several nights together. [Illegible] *but like stinking smoke. The* dose *as much as will cover a shilling.*

Griping the Belly

Mint or peneroyal water, Milk hott with pepper, green or dry Ginger, Sothern wood. Heat hott, & apply it to the Navel, or belly. Wormwood or Camomile used in like manner. If Griping be with costiveness, use a Clyster. If it be with a loosenes, then use purging

---

42. That is, the ligature will be sloughed during healing. Only aneurysms in superficial vessels can be ligated in this way.

43. Urethral discharge was to be treated with a remedy made from the pizzle, or penis, of an ox, an application of the doctrine of *similia similibus curantur* (like things are cured by like things).

potions downwards, as Manna, Roses or the like & spoonfull of Dock seed boyld in beer.

Belly Bound

Cassia dissolved in Chicken broth, 1 oz. Or anoint with Juice of Sothernwood. Or Rx. Aloes as much as a hazel nut. Beat together with 8 or 9 Raysons of the Sune stoned, roule (roll) in Pills & so take it fasting. [Page 65]
Let the patient eat a roasted Apple going to bed mixed with butter & Ginger. Or take an Onion, make an hole therein & fill it with pure honey & a little of Pulp of Coloquintida. Roast it & lay to the navel. It will help.

Another

Rx. Sena & white Tartar, of each 1 oz.; Cinnamon, Galingal, 1 dram; Diagridum, 2 drams. In fine powder searse them; the Dose, 1 dram in whey.

Another

Rx. Mechoacan (not of N.E. [New England]), 2 oz.; Gentian, 1 oz.; Diagridium, gr. (grains) 12; in powder. The Dose in whey, 1 dram.

Belly, looseness long continued

Mithridate or Treacle mixed with Conserve of red Roses. Take morning & E[vening]; the quantity of a Nutmeg.

Another

The powder of white thorn haws, the stones being pickt out. Let the patient eat it in thin broth made of mutton or Veale. It will stay the lask. Or powder of Bramble buds boyld in broth. Or take an Apple & empty out the Core, & fill the empty place with beeswax & roast the apple & eat it.

A quince is better. Take this for a sure rule, that if binding things do not presently help in a looseness then you must use purging to purge away the cause.

To purge the Belly of Children and to Kill the Worms

Rx. The pulp of Coloquintida, 1 scruple & infuse the same in pure Sallot oyl for the space of 24 hours, or else infuse of Aloes [Page 66] cicatrine, 2 scruples in warm Sallot oyl and annoint the child's navel over night when he goes to bed with either of these. The same will make the belly loose & kill the worm.

Boyls of Felons

Smallage, rue, sage, mixed with Leven (leaven, yeast) or Fetherfew with leven or yest. F. Empl. Or garden snails with the shells stampt to a plaister. Or Mithridates with yolk of an Egg. F. Empl. Will draw out the soar & heale it.

Blood Flux

The dissease is known by long avoiding (voiding) of blood by stoole or siege. Rx. Milk a pint, water a pint. Let them boyl together to a pint. Drink no other drink. If it continue, then if the patient be able open a Veine in the arm. Or Rhubarb well torrified at the fire. Or 1 dram in Conserve of red roses or Mechoachan, to children 1 scruple. Or 1 or 1½ dram to them of age. Or Syr. of Roses solutive. The use of Clysters after the decoctions of plantain, purslane, endive, barberry.

To take away the pains

Often lick sallet oyl & sugar boyld together, or fresh butter, also goats or hogs fat, or fat of foul (fowl) used in Clysters. A Clyster made of sheeps head broth, the flesh falling from the bones. If paine be very great, Philonium Romanum or Laudanum [Page 67] or opium, 4 gr., dissolved in Clysters.

Collected out of the Generall practise.[44]

Stench of Arm Pitts

If it continue long a sure sign of incidant (incident, falling) palsy. Purge; let blood; bath with odoriferous herbs as Mint, Melilot, Lavender. Foment the arm pits & whole body with annis, Cumarin, roses, &c. If it escoriate the place & skin, bath with warm water & strew on powder of Allom. Marmalade with spices expells all stench.

Chaps in hands

Rx. Sallade oyl, or oyl of Roses & wax melted together. F. Ungt. Or oyle of Roses, white wax, mastic, frankencse (frankincense) & hens greese. F. Ungt.

Scabby Hands

Rx. Gum. Tragacanth dissolved in rose water & rub the hands, or sweet butter, turpentine, wash together certain times with Vinegar. Temper it with 2 oz. of Salt & Cerus 3 drams & wash with it. Vid. Genll Practise Page 522.[45]

Bleeding at Nose

Lint made into tents, dipped in Vinegar, stuffed up the Nose. Vinegar Clouts to the Codds & the Pulse one (on) both Wrists, or a Cupping glass to the Navil with a great flame or Bole [of] wine Vinegar, white of egge, Plaisters thereof to the temples. Hoggs dung, hot from the hogg, with Sugar applyed or frankincense, Aloes, hairs of a Hare, white of a Egg, mixed & applyed, or Bole [of] Dragons Blood, franc. (frankincense), Aloes. F. Pulvis. [Page 68] Or hold Lips of the Wound with a finger till blood be clotted. Or apply a

---

44. *The General Practise of Physicke* by Christopher Wirtzung. Palmer does not identify the edition he used. Editions of the translation appeared in 16—?, 1605, 1617, and 1654.

45. Apparently, quotation from *The General Practice* ends here.

peice of Sal [illegible] or apply white or red Lead in powder, or a peice of an ould Hatt.

Biting of Doggs, horses, Swine etc.

Press the blood out of the wound. Blood letting, Purging, sometimes a dehesind (dehiscent) made of clay & Vinegar above the wound. Wound kept open & brought to suppuration. *If poison* be feared, use butter, Treacle, ol. Roses, unguent Basilicon. F. medicine & apply it. On a bite not venomous, use mallows, Camomile, wormwood. Soft boyle or mix an Egg, butter, safron, ol. Ros., ol. Viol. & apply them.

For Suppuration

Rx. powder of Myrh, Aloes, of each 1 dram; with honey or Roses, F. Ungt. If danger of a gangreen, look to the signs & cure of a Gangreen.

Biting of Venemous Beasts

First the Poison must be lett or drawn out. Cupping Glasses with Scarrification or take hens or Pigeons cut in the middle alive & apply hott to the wound for 6 or 8 hours.[46] If the Danger be great & the place [Page 69] bitten not full of Nerves, cutt out the flesh round about the bitten. Mix wine or Vinegar with Treacle, & wash the wound, then open the wound & cause it to bleed plentifully. Apply to it a roasted Onion with Salt & rue bruised, or Pigeons dung, or hens dung, sod with [illegible] of beer to draw out the remainder of the poison. If the Wound be already inflamed, the part inflamed must be deeply scarrifyed & bleed plentifully, after which apply the next foregoing Medicines. After the poyson is drawn forth, the inflamation or swelling eased, The Cure is easy, with Ungt. Basilicon & Turpentine &c.

46. An application of the ancient doctrine of animal transference. The body of a freshly killed animal when applied to the wound was believed to draw out the poison.

Another way of curing. First open the wound to cause it to bleed; after apply powder of Virginia Snakeweed with Treacle & give the patient of the same in Wine to drink. Apply to the wound garlic, Mithridate, powder of Snakeweed. *To prevent* Serpents biting, take Juice of Radish roots & annoint the hands therewith & the smell thereof will not only cause them to forbear biting, but be ready to die though you take them up in your hands.

Biting of a Mad Dogge

The first direction before concerning biting is available for this. Another. Rx. Leaves of Rue, Verveine, Sage, Plantaine, polipod. Wormwood, Mints, Mugwort, Balm, bettony, [St.] Johnswort of equal weight & they are best gathered in June & dryed in the shade. [Page 70] Beat [illegible] or some of them to powder and give 2 oz. in a spoon with double sugar, else in drink, broth, butter, honey every day for 3: or 4 dayes together. If it be long after the biting and the patient becomes fearfull of water, in the mean time the wound must be fomented 2 or 3 times a day, with wine, or honey water & some of the former powder. After this your ordinary wound oyntmt will cure it.

Another Rx. White onions N[umber] 3; make them hollow, & fill up the hollow with Treacle set on the Covers. Roast them on the Coals till they be soft, then stamp them & straine them through a Scarfe. Adde pulv. utriusque Aristioloch, 2 drams; Galb. (gallbanum), Bdell[ium], Myrrh, of each 2 oz.; pulv. Cancer fluv., 6 drams; mix. F. Cataplasm.

Another Rx. Galbanum Sa., Opop. (opoponax), Ass. fet. (asafoetida), Fat, Myr. piperis (Myrtus piperis), Sulph(ur), of each ½ oz.; Calamint, ½ oz.; Stercus Columbini, Anatis, each 2 oz. Dissolve gums in white wine, mix them with honey & ould oyl. F. Emplastr.

Against all biting, a Plaister

Rx. Sapuma (spuma) Argenti, Cerussa, of each 1 lb.; ol[eum] veteris lib. q.s.; wax, 2 oz.; ammoniacum, 4 oz.; galbanum, 4 oz.

Boyl the Coruss (cerussa), Litherge (litharge) & oyl till they be cleaving to your hands, then dissolve the gumms & ad them.

Bruises

[Page 71] If the bruise be great, let a vein be opened, on the contrary (opposite) part, or else let Ligatures be used. Also use repellent for Medicines as oyl of Roses, or the white of eggs alone. Next the clottered blood must be dissolved & scattered. If the bruises be inward—
Rx. Rhubarb trit[urated], 2 oz.; mumme, ¹/₂ oz.; rubia majoris, 2 oz.; Syr. de ros. sicc., ¹/₂ oz. F. Potio. Aliud: Rx. Terra sigillata rubia tinct., Mumme, symphite, of each 1 scruple; Rhubarb trit., 1 scruple. Mix them cum aqua pastoris burs. Plantaginis.

For clottered under the Skin

If it be over all the body or in many parts thereof, take a sheeps skin newly pluckt of from the Sheeps back & sprinckle it with powder of water Cresses & small beaten salt & lap it about the patient & let him sweat in it.[47]

For Blood clottered in some one part

Rx. Decoctions of Camomile, Wormwood, Cleonin & bath the part therein, or take barly Meale & Calamint & make a Pultis.

For one bruised by a fall

Stone pitch or Rosin beaten small, mixed with white wine & drink it cold. Or Spermaceti taken inwardly & hott apply'd outwardly. [Page 72]

Burning & Scaldings

Ungt. Basilicon takes out the fire presently. If the place be raw, ungu[entum] album or the juice of a brake root, mixt with Cream or

---

47. Again, the doctrine of animal transference. The clots were expected to move from the human skin to the skin of the sheep.

the oyl of Eggs. Or oyntment made of Mall[ows], plantain, night shade, Mulleine, Roses, Henbane, any of these or any other cold herb, or oyntment of Populeon, or oyl boyled out of beaten pumpion (pumpkin) seeds.

Burning with Gunpowder

Wash the place with brine & apply Clouts wet therein, or the juice of houseleeck mixt with the white of eggs. Or Goose dung fryed with fresh butter till the butter be almost consumed; strain it out and anoynt 3: times a day & dip linnen Cloths in the oyntment & apply them. This will cure all sorts of burnings [even] though with Gun-powder.

Rx. Beeswax, mutton, suet & the green mold that grows on the backside of houses on the wall, scraped off on a rainy day & stewed together takes out the fire & heals any burn or scald.[48] Strain it out when boyled together. It makes an excellent green salve. Probat. est.

A sup of suety broth with ale. Eat nothing but curd with this. [Page 73]

Canker in the nose, throat &c to cure

Rx. Vitriol alb., 1 oz., burnt to powder; Alum, burnt, ¹/₂ oz.; mixed together, blow up the nostrils & mixed with honey & rubbed on the palate of the mouth. It is good to mix with it the poudr of holly leaves burnt to ashes. *The nostrils rubbed with this brings down the cankers on lips.*[Page 74]

Cancers

A Canser is a hard unequal round Venemous humour, blackish of Colour, suddenly encreasing & very painfull & wearing to the patient without intermission, bred of burnt choler. The humour is salt in tast. It may grow in any part of the body, especially in the face, lips, ears & womens brests that lack their natural sicknes & it is hardly (with difficulty) cured. Inward Cancers admit no cure, nor those that

48. The therapeutic use of mold long antedated the discovery of penicillin.

are inveterate, unless they be cured by incision or burning. Those persons are most subject to them that have been accustomed to the Hemorroids & lost the benefit thereof.

The Diet must be sparing & of sutable juice. Open a Veine if the age & strength suffer (permit). It must be salved out, burnt out, or cut out by the roots. With other remedys, often purging & letting blood are to be used. Some have affirmed that a Diet drink constantly taken of Lignum vitae wood or bark has cured a Cancer, but it has been (if so) by changing the natur of the humour & converting a Salt humour into a sweet humour. Some have been cured by Verdigrease Copperas, Alum boyld in Smiths water & so wash often. Vid. Indian Med [icine] for Cancer in the Vad. Mecum with Deers lether Covers.

A *Cancer Ulcerate*

is a round tumorous ulcer, horrible stincking, [Page 75] with the Lips of it thick & hard, knotty, turned under, strutting (swelling, bulging) upward & hollow, the colour blackish & obscure, with Veines in the Circuit of the Ulcer full of Melancholly blood, the cause thereof, the matter flowing out thin, watrish, black or yellow, evil savouring.

Prognosticks

If in the Veins, Sinews & bones is hardly cured. It must be fetcht out by roots, by Diet, bleeding & purging. Cut it wholly away with an incision Knife, presse the thick blood out of the Veines nere to it that it may flow forth again, joyn the lips of the ulcer togeth[er] & go forward to cure it as other ulcers. Some consume it with a Cautery; with Caustick Medicine it may be done as with arsenic sublimate, used warily, but then the places about it must be defended with ung. de bolo from inflammation. After[ward] procure the falling away [of] the Eskar as in other ulcers.

Rx. Rock Allum, $^{1}/_{2}$ oz.; verdigrease, 3 drams. Use this water with Syringe. Give the patient broth of red Coleworts 3 times a day. *Many medicines* that are cooling and prescribed, but I fear it doth drive away the humour to some other part.[49] Some have used in the beginning

49. An explanation for what is now called metastasis.

of a Cancer oyl of Cloves that has eaten it away. To Know whether a Cancer be in the flesh, sinews, or bone, mix honey and the Gaule of a Goat together & anoint the place with it. If it be in the flesh, thick will issue forth; if it be [Page 76] in the bone, water; if it be in the Sinew, thin water. Many other things are used by Authors for Cancer but to little purpose. Some make Medicine for a Cancer with oyl & spirit of Vitriol commix tog[ether] and so eat it out, & to heale it boyl tobacco in white wine Vinegar & add Sallat oyl thereto.

Catarh or Rhumes

It is a great flux of Rhumes, & it some times is a hot rhume & some times a cold. Signes of a hot Catarh: if the Rhume be thin and sharp, the head hot, face & eyes red; if it excoriates the parts. If bitterness, or saltness, be perceived, Signs of a cold Catarh.

If the humour that doth distill be with out savour & not biting heviness about the eyes, then it is a cold Catarh.

Also the Causes that went before the Catarh do discover whether it was by any disorder in diet, or evil disposition of any part.

Cure of Cold Catarh

In young persons bleeding by a Veine is good. Take Mochoac, 1 dram, with Ginger (but not this of N.E.) (New England). Infuse a night in white wine, upon embers, & drink the wine fasting, Pil. Alaphangia or Cassia de agarico, or de Iliona cum agarico, mastic alone, eaten at night going to bed. Or take Nutmeg, 1 dram; mastic, Gum Arabic, 1/2 dram. With rose water make [Page 77] Troches. Or Conserve of red Roses, 2 oz.; Nutmegs, 1 scruple; white frankincense, 2 scruples; with Syr. of dry roses, F. Elect. Take as much as a Walnut going to bed. When as the Catarh has continued long, infusion of China, Guajacum, Sassafras, Sarsaparilla, to help against a cold Catarh. Fumes is bedward[50] made with Franckincense, Cinnamon, Sage, Marjoram, rosemary.

---

50. That is, at bedtime expose the patient to the fumes of the following.

To cure a Hot Catarhe

Purg(atives) of Manna, Rhubarb, Syr. Roses, or Pil. Aurea or Arabic are useful. Clysters, washing hands before meals. A Plaster of Pigeons dung. Thapsia was used by Galen. A Seton in the Neck, or Pil. de Cynagloss., from 6 grains to 1 scruple, at going to bed.

To help a Catarh, Strangling that threatens, sharp Clysters, open a Veine, Cupping Glass to Arms, thighs, also purging Medicines, Fumes, Mastic, Frankincense, Amber, Smoke of Rope, Vinegar poured upon a hot stone, the Gum Taccamahacca dissolved with a hot Iron & put on a Cloth & applyed to the temples, some times powder of Amber, Frankincense & mastick, white of an egge & rose water applyed to temples is available but this stop so strongly therefore it must be taken away after an hour or two & renewed again. The neck is to be anoynted with oil of amber. Also take of Euphorbium & wax & make a Cerat for the Crown of the head after it is shorn. [Page 78]

Or Rx. Nigella torrifyed, $1/2$ oz.; Mustard Seed, 3 drams; Frankincense & Mastic, $1^{1}/_{2}$ drams; pigeon dung, barly meals, of each $1/2$ oz.; Oximel simplex, q.s. F.E. [mplastrum] for the Crown of the Head. Take a little leaven, fatt, figgs, six Cantharides, the Heads and wings being clipt off, & with Vinegar of Squills make a mass, but take it off after 6 hours. Also the Loch. of squills, with Oximel, bole Armoniack is to be given. Also remember that in case of long continued Catarrhe, the body be purged once a month, a little before the New-Moon, especially if the body be subject to costiveness. Also a seton in the Arms is very needfull in this case. Also in this case fennel seed, Anniseed, Cummons, Coriander, with a little sugar dissolved & hardned are good after meals. Let the Diet be sparing, easy of Digestion, dry, solid food, little spoon meats, their suppers little or none at all. Consider the causes of this Rheume whether it do not come from the cold & weak temper of the Stomach, or from the weake temper of the Liver that doth not digest the Chilus (chyle) into good blood. See the [diagnostic] signs of either in their proper places.

Rx. Agarici albi, $1^{1}/_{2}$ oz.; Species Diambre, $1/2$ oz.; Diaireos Solomon, 1 dram; Spec(ies) Diatragacanthi, 4 scruples; Polopodii Quercini, 1 oz. Omnia in pulverus redacta cum saccaro incorporentur ad placit.[51] This is excellent for a Catarrhe falling upon the Lungs. [Page 79]

Chollick & Cure

It hath the Name because it is seated in the Gutt Colon. It is caused of wind, or the hardnes of excrements, or by the stone or of Worms. Sometimes by hot humours, sometimes of cold & thick humours, & sometimes by the maligning of humours. Windines of the stomach is to be distinguished from the Chollick, for the paine of the Stomach is always above the Navel & reacheth to the spine bone, between the shoulders & is eased with belching & vomiting, which is not in the Chollick, which is seated under the Navel beginning about the right Kidney & so passeth to the Liver, & usually causeth Vomiting.

The Chollick differs from the Stone in the Kidneys because the Chollick is most in the former parts & the stone in the hinder parts in the Kidneys & Ureters. The Chollick runs from part to part but the stone paine abides constantly in the same place, as Kidneys & thighs. In the Stone the Urine is full of small gravel or very clere.

Cure

Begin with Clysters, mallows, Parietory, camomile flours, fenegreek, oyl of Sweet almonds, Camole [camomile?], Dill, hens fat or goose fatt. Also infusion of camomile and dill is excellent to be drunk in this case.

If the wether be could & the cause and matter of the dissease be hot, use oyl of violets, oyl of Roses with the yolks of eggs, also Milk. Apply all in a blader [Page 80] or in linnen Cloths for a fomentation. If Paine be in extremity use Narcotiques, as Philonium Romanum, requies Nicolais, of either 1/2 dram with infusion of chamomile flours. Also Laudanum Opiatum given in 2 grains or 4 grains at once, only let these Narcotiques be used while the patient hath some strength

---

51. Everything is reduced to powder with sugar added according to taste. The Latin is faulty.

& not when he is very weake. Also these Narcotiques are excellent in Clysters, as Rx. decoction of Chamomile flour, 1 lb.; Philonium Romanum or requies Nicolais, ½ oz.; ol. Amigd. dulc. F. Clyster. Some things give ease by secret qualities. Rx. dry toasted wheat bread; soak it in Malmsey or sweet wine. Cast Lavender flours on the toast, bind it to the Navil, as hot as may be, till it be cold, then another, it never faileth. It will do without the Lavender flours. Also Wolves white dung with a little salt & peper in white wine being drunk is very good. Also the dry gutts of wolves being at the Navil is good. Stones of horses in powder with Sack & Anniseed is excellent. When Clysters help not in the Cholick, a gentle purge of manna. Rx. Manna, 1½ oz.; ol. Amigd. dulc., 1½ oz. in fat hen's broth. Or make a plaister thus.

Rx. Empl[astrum] De baccis Lauri, Empl. de melilot, of each 2 oz.; cum ol. camom. & Ruta. F. Empl. If wind only cause the chollick, a hot brick into a linnen cloth dipped in wine & layd to the Navil will help.

The diet in the Chollick must be opening & [Page 81] such as may scatter wind. Garlick is good, raw or roasted.

The Drink should be white wine, or water & honey boyled together.

The Chollick that cometh of Wormes

Sometimes young persons are grieviously tormented with this kind of cholick & continual fever & other evident signs of worms. Give Aloes in the pap of an Apple, Clysters of New Milk & Sugar. Apply to the Navel Aloes, Honey & turpentine plaister wise to the Navel, or the Gaul of an Ox & wormwood to the Navel.

Chollick caus'd of thick & Viscous humours in the Gutts sticking thereto

This Paine is like a stake stuck in the Gutts or an Augur boring in the belly, fastened in some part.

THE CURE

Emollient Clysters made of Rue, Beets, Caraway seeds; add to it Diacatholicon & Hiera, of each ½ oz.; Ol. Cham. [chamomile] & Ruta, ½ oz. Make thereof a Clyster. Purge with mel rosarum solut.

or Hira simplex, or Pills of Mastick, or Pills of Benedicta laxativa made up with turpentine. Garlick eaten is good in this case. Castor often taken in Hydromel is good. The belly is to be anoynted with oyl of sweet Almonds, or oyl of Chamomile, or Dill, or Bayes. [Page 82]

Consumption

It is to be considered in the beginning, or in the termination & extremity thereof. It may be considered as the whole body is wasting, or some part of it. A consumption of the whole body is to be considered, as the whole body is lean & wasted & gets no good by nourishing things.

Signs. The Temples are fallen, the Eyes are sunk into the head, nose sharp, Cheek-bones stick out. The belly is fallen & empty & heavines is in the whole body.

The Causes are many. Sometimes obstructions, sometimes the humidum radicale or Calor naturalis is spent, some-times from salt Rhumes, some-times from outward Causes, & divers other diseases & frequently with a Cough that is continuing.

Cure

Keep from Costiveness, from any Disquietments, oppression by hard labours. Such drink & food as bread (breed) much blood & spirits. As much oyle Olive, honey, new-milk, Egges, roasted meats that are fatt. Sweet wines, much strong bear or Ale, Jellys of Fowl &c., Raisins, Pruans, Figgs, & much change of Diet.

MUTTON BERE THUS MADE

Take all the fat principle parts of a Sheep, boyl them all to peices, that the flesh fall from the bones. Then strain it out & make a bushell of bear with a bushell of malt & this Mutton broth. Mash it & order it as other bere. Drink of it 4 or 5 times a day. [Page 83]

Consumption of some parts only

As the arms or Leggs, look carefully to the cause. Some times it comes by streight (strait) binding; by a swelling by a bone out of

...or in linnen Cloth &c ———————————

If paine be ... extreamely use Narcotiques,
as Philonium Romanum, requies Nicolai;
of either ʒ. ℥ ℈ of Chamomile flours,
also Laudanum Opiatum given in gr. ii or
grains at once, only let these Narcotiques
be used while ye patient hath ... some ...
... not when he is very weake. also these
Narcotiques are excellent in Clysters,
as ℞ decoction of Chamomile flours lb j.
Philonium Romanum or requies Nicolai
℥ss. ol. Amigd: dulc. F. Clyster. some
things give ease by secret qualities ———
℞ dry toasted wheat bread, soak it in
Malmsey or sweet wine, cast Lavender
flours on ye toast, bind it to ye Navil, as
hot as may be, till it be cold, then another, it never faileth. it will do without ye
Lavender flours. Also Wolves white dung wth a
little salt & pepper in white wine being drōk
is very good. also ye dry gutts of wolves hāg
at ye Navil is good.
Stones of horses in powder ℈ j. each wth ...
is excellent. when Clysters helps not in
Cholick, a gentle purge of manna
℞ Manna ℥ ij. ol. Amigd. dulciū ℥ j.
in fat hens broth. or make a glaister take
℞ Empl. de baccis Lauri Empl. de ...
ana ℥ij. cū ol. cemoni. & Rub ... Empl.
If wind only cause ye chollick, a hot brick ...
into a linnen cloth dipped in wine & layd to ye
Navil will helpe. ———————
The hot ... chollick must be ...

_____

The Drink should be white wine, or water &
honey boyl'd together. y.̃ chollick y.̃ cometh of
stomack. some times young persons are grievou-
sly tormented of this kind of cholick, & continual
now & y.̃ vicisi—— agues of worms.
Give Aloes in y.̃ pap of an Apple, Clysters of
New Milk & sugar apply to y.̃ Navel Aloes
honey & turpentine plaister wise to y.̃ Navel
or y.̃ Gaul of an Ox & wormwood to y.̃ Navel.

C. Chollick caused of thick & C.
Viscous humours in y.̃ Gutts
Sticking thereto.

This Paine is like a stake stuck in y.̃ Gutts
or an Augur boring in y.̃ belly fastned in
some part. ~~~~~~~~~

The Cure.

Emollient Clysters, made of Rue Betts
Caraway seeds, add to it Diacatholicon &
Hiera, ana ℥ss. Ol. Cham. & Rute ℥ss.
mak: thereof a Clyster, purge w.̃ Mel Rosar̄u
solut. or Hiera simplex, or Pills of mastick,
or Pills of Benedicta laxatira, made up w.̃ turpentine. garlick eaton is good in this case.
Castor often taken in Hydromel is good, the
belly is to be anoynted with oyl of sweet Almonds, or oyl of Chamomile, or Dill or Bayes.

place; sometimes by a wound, by the cutting of a great Veine or Artery, then it is incurable. Otherwise our endeavour must be to draw blood & spirits to the part by unctions & hand frictions, often every day, till the part be increased again. Make this Oyl.[52] [Rx. Tips of Juniperus sabina, leaf of levistici, of each 2 minims; camomile flowers, 2 parts. All are cut up & finely divided. Add oleum laurini & lilioni, as much as necessary. Mix all with hog's fat (recommended is that which is extracted from a red hog), 4 oz.; alcohol, 2 oz. Let all this be done quickly before the moisture is consumed and squeezed out. Add oil of spike or ditto of juniper berries, 2 drams; add powdered black mustard seed, ½ oz.; of pyrethrum roots, 3 drams; long or round pepper of Zanzibar, 2 drams; beeswax as necessary. Make an unguent. Add the fat of the horse, dog, bear, fox, and butter. Item, oil of earthworm, beaver, or elephant, 2 lb.]

Also, it is good to anoynt the part with the blood of a Calf, adding some peper to it. Also it is powerful to thrust the consumed part into the body of an ox or Cow newly killed, to do it often.[53] Baths of hot herbs are profitable, being used before unction.

Cough

It comes sometimes from a mean distemper of heat or could, sometimes from Rhume, hot or cold, that falls up on the lungs, or the Arteria Aspera, from an ulcer in the lungs, from a Pleurisy, from inflammation of the liver & spleen, as in the dropsy of Smoak or Dust. But note that if a Cough do continue many months, it is dangerous, especially to women with child, & is the death of many of them. Avoid costivenes or whatsoever causeth it, as cheese. Keep to a dry diet that is fat, drinks made of Lignum Vitae wood [Page 84] and Elecampane & Anise seed. Liquorice or the wood alone is the only remedy above all others to any that have it with a tickling in the throat. Take the small saw dust or very small chipps of the

---

52. The following passage in square brackets has been translated from Palmer's Latin.

53. An application of the theory of animal transference.

wood. Boyl it alone or with other things in a bottle of fair water to a quart. Drink 3 or 4 spoon fulls of this drink 4 or 5 times a day, provided the body be not costive. For a tickling Cough, for a Salt Rhume, or Phlegm, for women with Child that have a Cough, I think there is not the like medicine. *A charm by God's blessing. I have oft feared, given, healed, and gained thereby for a* cough. *But for* myself, *mean and bitter fluids. This from Dr. Fuller.*[54]

An Excellent medicine for Cough In Children

Rx. Anniseed, 1 lb.; Liquorice, ½ lb. Beat the seed small & also beat or shread the Liquorice very small. Then Distill it with an Alembick, having added about 4 or 5 quarts of water, & first let it steep 24 hours, & then Distill off the water with a slow fire till the tast of the Anniseed & Liquorice be almost gone. Then separate your oyl of Anniseed that is on the top of the water, take off the lembeck (alembic), & strain out all the liquor that is in your pot through a fine hair sieve, & boyl up this water with Sugar, till it come to the thicknes of thick honey. This is better liquorice juice than the Apothecarys make, excellent for the Cough, a little taken at a time, several times a day, [Page 85] for Young or ould, & for Young or ould mix a few drops of the oyl with Liquorice juice. But for infants that cannot take other medicine, take the distilled water that the oyl was taken off from. Take that clear thin water, after the oyl is separate, & mix ½ lb. of Sugar to a pint of the water, & so keep it for use. Give a Child a spoon full at a time, often.

Many Medicines are made for a Cough of Rosemary, sage, Peneroyal, Hysop wine, Alocampane (Elecampane), scabious, fennel, mouse ear, maiden hair, figgs, raisens, these or any of them. New milk boyld with sugar & butter for many nights together. Sugarcandy. Cough of a thin Rhume, use such things as are spoken of for a Catarrh. Take Cloves & Mace, 2 or 3 penny worth; bay-salt, a handfull, dryed at the fire; Cumin & Frankencence, 1 oz.; Sage, 1 minim. Take all these & beat them well together. Put them in a

---

54. One of Palmer's more cryptic shorthand passages. He seems to be apologizing for the use of a cough remedy that he believes is effective but also considers to be a charm.

Linnen bagg, as long and as broad as the hand, quilt in this Powder, & lay it to the mould of the Head. Warm it every morning & evening.

To Cure the Cough from a hott and thin Rhume

Juice of Liquorice & white starch, also Conserve of Roses & Violets, with Bole Armoniack mixed and good. Or Rx. Barly, ½ minim; four cold seeds, 1 dram; white poppy, 2 drams; Liquorice, 1½ drams; jujubes, ten in number. Coquin s.q.; aqu. Colat., 10 oz. Add Syr. Violets & Jujubes, do (ditto) [Syr.] papaveri, 2 oz.: use it at several doses. Also use this powder. Rx. white starch, 2 drams: bole Armoniack, 1 oz.; Gum Arabick, Gum tragacanth, 2 drams. Liquorice powder, 1 oz.; sugar candy, ½ oz. Mingle these & take each [Page 86] morning fasting as much as will ly upon a shilling. If there be danger of breaking the inward vessels by the Vehemency of Coughing, use Treacle, Phylonium Romanum, Pil. de Cynaglos., Laud. Opiatum.

To Cure the Cough Coming of Phlegmatick Humours

After the use of some gentle purge, or Pills, then the Syrup of Maiden-hair, Hyssop & Liquorice, Oximel either simple or compound, or of squills with the water of Hysop or maiden hair, scabious &c. Rx. Figgs, N.X.; Liquorice & Anniseed, Hysop. Make an infusion. Use Loch sanum or Loch de pulmone Vulpis.

For an Ould Cough

Rx. Honey and butter, of each 4 oz. Cummin seed in pouder, 1 dram. Mix the butter with the honey dispumed (despumed), heat them & then mix them together for the patient. Or take Cumin, peper & Nettle seed; mix 1 oz. of each with a pint of clarifyed honey. Or take Elecampane roots, Hysop, maiden hair, Carduus, the Cordial flours, Liquorice, Anniseed, all these in pouder; figgs, 8 in number. Let all these be set in an earthen pott in an oven, the ingredients covered over with honey that is clarifyed. Bake it with a batch of bread, & let the patient take a spoonfull M[orning] & evening, also when the matter of the Cough is very thick & tough.

[Rx] Coltsfoot, peneroyal, parsly; infuse them in honey, a pint; of Vinegar, half a pint; boyl these with a gentle fire, strain them, adding decoction of pennyroyal a pint. Add mithridate or Treacle, 1½ oz. Give a spoonfull of this in the morning & before supper. To the same thou mayest add [Page 87] Syrup of Hysop or Loch de pino.

A POWDER FOR THIS COUGH

Rx. Powder of Liquorice, 3 drams; Anniseed & Fennel, of each 1½ dram; the species of Diatragacanth frigidi, 1 dram; species Diaireos Simplex, ½ dram; Flos sulphuris, 2 scruples; Fox lungs, 2 scruples; White sugar candy, 1½ oz. Make a powder & take as much fasting as will ly upon a shilling.

Chin Cough

Bath the soals of the Feet with warm hoggs fatt going to bed, wrap them up warm, in cloths. Or powder of a dryed Mouse drunk in ale, or take parsly juice, pouder of Cummin, womens milk, mix them & give the Child to drink. Make this oyntment for the stomach. Rx seed of Hemp or Flax & Fenucrik (fenugreek); seeth these in fair water. Add fresh butter, Capon fatt, oyl of white Lillys & oyl of sweet Almonds, of each 2 drams; wax q.s. F. ung.

Or take the muscilage or seeds of hemp & flax & Fenugreek & add to the former oyls. Or take of white starch, 1 oz. Dissolve it in milk, boyl to the form of a Pultis, ad fresh butter & sugar, and being could eat it. Or take Turpentine, yolk of an egge, fresh butter & hony & mix them for use. Or take Sulphur, 1 oz.; orice (orris), ½ dram; Sugar candy, 1½ oz.; take this with a soft egge or Juniper berrys & Hysop boyled in wine. Cures the cough in children. So doth distilled water of Hysop. Item, a few drops of the oyl of Hysop mixed with Sugar & the stomach about the Pitt of it with the oyl anointed, 3 or 4 drops at a time. Also Diacodium & Syr. of Poppy is gracious in this case, being licked. Also popy water with sugar Candy given at going to bed. Consider [Page 88] the Causes: In a hott cause annoynt the brest with oyl of Violets, oyl of sweet Almons, fresh butter, hens fatt, the Muscilage of the Seed Psyllium. In a Cold Cause, oyl of land Lyllys, Psyllium Muscilage of Linseed, Fennugreek, Orrias. Saffron, a little wax for an ointmt. for the brest.

Also, Onions & Garlic mixed with butter, being well roasted, apply'd to the brest, with the feet with warm water bed ward.

Cough of the Lungs

In the beginning the disease is cured, but long continued it is not. If the Lungs be ulcerated in the beginning,
Rx. Liquorice, Orrice, Elocampane in pouder, make into Pills with Pix liquida. Take 4 every morning fasting. Conserve of Red Roses with Bole Armoniac & olibanum & Syr. Myrtles. F. Elect. Take the quantity of a great Nutmeg every Night.
Or make an infusion of Raisins, Anniseed figgs, Maiden hair, sugar; take of this often. But if anything does good in this case, it must be such medicines as are healing, cleansing & increase good blood & spirits & cleanse by Urine, & keep the body from Costiveness & procure rest.

A Could

Before sleep after a Could is taken, a spoon full of Sallet oyl with Sack or posset ale. If it have taken possession of the body, it cause fevers & aches & in the beginning. Take a Vomit or take Hysop, Peneroyal, Anniseed, Liquorice, Ginger, Figgs. F. an infusion in ale. Sweeten it with sugar. Take often several dayes together. [Page 89]

When a Could hath stopped the Nose and Head

Fill your Mouth with water & then snuff up the juice of Primrose into your Nose. Keep warm. When a Flux of Rhume is caused by a Could, let the sick Person (saith Mr. Cheney) dip his head into a bason of could water, 2 or 3 times. This is not good for Women, nor in fevers.

To open the Pipes stopped with a Could

Rx. Endive, Succory, Parsly, Fennel, borage, hop, Time, Peneroyal, Germander, Nep (*Nepeta*), F. an infusion in water. Ad good wine, Vinegar & sugar. Or else Rx of Grap water, a pint; as much of stale Ale; Sugar Candy, 1 oz., being boyld together slowly a little while. Add a bruised stick of Liquorice at one end, dip it into the liquor & suck the Juice from the stick.

Choler to cure & purge it away especially from the Stomach

Signs hereof are loathing Food, bitternes in the mouth, of *smoke*, sence of Gnawing in the Stomach. Sometimes Vomiting, Choler. For this case, Vomits of Crocus Metallorum, Purges of rubarb, manna. Or else take of the Roots of Munks Rubarb, thin sliced, Mints, Wormwood; steep them in ale or strong beer a night. Take of it fasting for several dayes together, betimes in the morning, especially in the spring. [Page 90]

Corns to Cure

Pare them neat, then put into the hole of the Corn a little sublimed Mercury & so close bind it up for a while. Or else a plaister of Galbanum or the inward part of a figg mixt with Verdegrease (verdigris). Or take Turpentine & red wax; boyl together & apply the same. Or a Plaister of Rosin wax oyl, Bole; keep it so till the Corn be destroyed & change it oft.

Cramp

Every night when you goe to bed smell to your fingars aftar you have picked the stincking sweat that is between yor toes. This will help without fail for an ordinary Cramp. When Convulsions are strong, bleeding or applying cupping glasses with scarification to a remote part, Strong Clysters, rubbing the neck with a warm cloth. Apply to the pt. (part) oyl of foxes, Castor or earthworms or oyl of turpentine, the wearing of a cramp ring, or a peice of the hoof of a Moose, made thin & small, & worn about the Neck, in a string. It is caused of wind that gathers into the part contracted. It.: the bone of a Raccoons pizzle. Probatum.

Convulsions

Powder of Castor, or spirit of Castor in an infusion of Sage, or Sage water, the decoction of Guajacum, Sassafras, Sassaparilla in Cramps, Convulsions, &c. First give a Clyster, then a Purge of Manna, Annoint nose, temples stomach with oyl of Amber, Sage, Rosemary &c.

Rx pulv. horse stooles as much as will ly upon a 6 pence for a man. prob. est. [Page 91 is blank. Page 92]

Dropsy

Signs are swelling of the feet, especially at night, difficult breathing, Palenes of the face & eyes, a Cough, sometimes a swelling in the legs, great thirst, lost appetite. Retention of stools, of sweat, of Vomiting, of the flowers &c. Small store of urine. 3 sorts of dropsy: Ascites, Hydrops, Timpanites. In Ascites the belly is swollen and full of water & sometimes the leggs & thighs, & the upper pts. of the body do dry away. The Cause is feebleness of the liver either through heat or cold, which hath not a sanguification or concoction but *turns her* moisture into water. Vid. General Practice of Physick.[55]

For a preparative Rx. Wormwood, Maiden hair. F. infusion in strong beer. Take it every morning fasting with 1 dram of Cream of Tartar. Purge with Pil Rhubarb, Mezereo, or Diaphenicon.

Or Rx. Mecoach (*Mechoacana*), 1 to 2 oz.; with Diagrid, 2 grains & a little Ginger, in powder fasting. Jallap, the dose from 1 scruple to 2 scruples in pulv. fasting. Juice of Elder roots or flowers, of Peach tree, dryed & boyled in broath, or Conserves of it, or Syrups, or Syr. of Elder berrys or Soldanella, or Sea Cabbage, ½ oz., with some Annis. Spice, 1 scruple. Sassafras roots & Guajacum continually taken is gracious in this Case; it purges by urine when the belly is full of water.

55. Wirtzung, 1617.

Rowel it in this wise.[56] Rx. Take up the skin between the fingers that is under the Navel half a handfull & peirce it with a great needle having a skein of white silk in it. Draw that silk through, applying of double cloths on the top of them drawing up & down the silk. You may in a few weeks draw out many Galls (gallons) of water this way without danger. Sometimes the water being sharp causeth an inflammation in the belly, but with cooling oyntments as Ung. Popul., succo fedi &c. [and] the inflammation may be holpen.

Oyntments for the Dropsy, ung. de Artanita, Agrippae, Ung. Martiatum, a Poultis of Pigeon's dung [Page 93] boyld in Ale, to the Navel applyd. Infusion of Bryony in water oft drunk fasting. The decoction of ash bark, in beer with parsly & fennel. Infusion of elder bark in beer or white wine. Strengthen the Liver. Remove the obstructions caused either by cold or heat with proper medicines. The Method of curing this Distemper consists in 3 points viz., the mollification of the indurate tumours in the bowels & other places, or to repel the peccant humours. Lastly drive out the same by stools and urine. *Therefore* drink seldom & little or *soberly and properly:* exercise reasonably. Sweat much, purge often, use clysters. Phlebotomy is forbidden, unless in women wanting the month. So move in Timpany. To move urine sweat and stoole, see more in General Practise of Physick, Pag. 404, 405. [Page 94 is blank. Page 95]

Deafnes

It hath several causes. If it be naturall from the Womb, it is not curable. If the inward membrane of the Skin called Timpanum be broken it is uncurable. If it come by reason of another Disease, when the other Disease is gone it will not long continue. That which is thick filth gathered in the Ears is curable. That which is caused by a cold, blood letting & purges. For strong remedys, sneezing pow-

---

56. *Rowel,* actually a veterinary term, meant to insert a seton, a strip of silk, linen, or cotton, in the flesh as a drain, in this case for fluid accumulated in the abdomen. This procedure is a form of counterirritation.

ders, or things that purge the Head by the Nose, Mastichatorys & things that avoid Rhume, Infusion of Rue, Rosemary or Marjoram, dropped into the Ears. Fair water injected 10 or 20 times into the ears. Gaule of living creatures especially with oyl of amber. Injected Carduus water & Hedghog fatt & liquid storax mixed together is exceeding powerfull. Or Ox gaul & she goat Urine, or childs mixt together, drop oft into the patients ear. Note that if deafness come by an ulcer in the ear, drop not in oyl or any fatt thing. Worm wood juice is good dropped into the deaf ear. Vid. General Practise.

Dysentery

This Disease or bloody flux is easily known by the bloodiness of the Seige. It hath usually a fever joyned with it & great torments of the bowells. It differs from all other Fluxes of blood, because that in the Dystentery there are other humours mixed with blood in the seige, also matter sometimes. If strength will endure, open a Veine, give torrifyed Rhubarb in plantain water, or Conserve of Roses, dose 1 dram. Mechoack, to Children 1 scruple, to others 1 dram or 1½ dram in fresh broath, barly water, Syr. of Roses solut[ion]. To it add pulp [of] tamarinds, 1 oz. Clysters of infusion of barly, Syr roses Solution, brown sugar or yolk of eggs, infusion of a hen, hony of roses. If pains be great use Laud[anum] opiatum. In Clysters, divers simples are good, as plantain, Comfry Nymphaea, sorrel, Crabgrass, bramble buds & all vulnary [Page 96] Herbs. So Bole, Terra sigillata, Lapis Hematites, Beeswax in a roasted apple, the Core taken out, Cervi Genitale exsiccatum & in pulvere redactum. Observe whether the blood that is voided be after the stool or on the outside of it, then it comes from the Hemorrhoids & doth come from the Spleen & is profitable.[57]

Observe whether the voiding of blood, following (follows) another white looseness or is mixed therewith. Observe whether the blood

57. Wirtzung's *General Practice of Physicke* taught that "melancholick blood" was carried by veins of the stomach and nearby spleen to hemorrhoidal veins that "expel the melancholick blood from them sometimes in great quantity, whereby nature is much unburthened, and getteth great health" (p. 304).

that is voided be like blood & phlegm mixed together & like the scrapings of gutts, or like bran mixed with blood, or whether it hath mixed colours, as green & the like, & great frequent motion to stool. Give syrup of Roses & whey, or manna or some other purge, for binding things will not do. I say in this case [*thus Mr. Fuller*] excrements of a man as green as copperas almost & purging prevailed most to his recovery. Observe that what you give to stay this skowring be always ministred before meals, for after meals binding medicines cause a sick body to scour the more. Froggs burnt to ashes stay blood. Vid. Genll. Practise. Pag. 353. [Page 97 is blank. Page 98]

Ears

Ulcers in the eares be caused by Impostumes and sometimes sharp humours in the Ears cause Impost. Sometimes the filth long continued do exulcerate them or from great blows or wounds not well cured. Some of the ulcers are in the inward parts, some in the outward parts, which make the cure more easy or difficult. The signs are the blood & filth that comes out of the Ears & when they come of Impostumes the matter flows abundantly at first, afterward is lessened. Besides there went before great paine & inflammation that are mitigated when the matter is voided, & in this trouble the paine is greater in the ear than in the head. But when filth comes from the Ears without an Impostume there is perceived an Itching about the Ear, & when the filth hath been evacuated, it gathers againe and again, unless it hath a free evacuation. It causeth giddiness & other symptoms. Such Ulcers as peirce to the bone of the Skull, are seldome or never cured.

Cure

Its good to wash the Ears with ould wine warm alone, or that wherein Roses or Leaves of Ivy have been boyled. After wash them with Hydromel, i.e., *water wherein honey hath been boyled*, or with the juice of wormwood, or Agrimony. Or the gaul of an hogg, wether, or ox may be dropped in. Or else take hony water & boyl in it the roots of white Hellebore adding Frankincense & Myrhh. Or take

hony and vinegar clarifyed & boyled, add verdegrees & drop this
into the ear. In ould ulcers Egyptiacum dissolved in *urine* is effectual
dropped into the ear, or else dissolved in a child's Urine. [Page 99]

Ears. Almons down[58]

Rx. Bole Armoniack, Fery Allom (ferric alum?), Nutmegs, mix
together. Take it oft in a day.

To Draw out Things fallen Into the Ears

They are things liquid or dry. If they be liquid as water, the way
is to drop in oyl, *as it* may be sucked out with Straw or Quill. If dry
things fall into the Ears *it's best way to force them out by sneezing with*
mouth and nose stopped. *If motes be fallen or carried into the* eyes drop
in the juice of wormwood or peach leaves, or also infuse roots of
white hellebore in wine, or mingle brimstone, chalk, honey & Vinegar. Drop in the ear.

Noise of the Eares

Cure is different according to diversity of Causes. If it come from
a hot distemper use the infusion of barly, lettice, Nymphea, popy
for a fomentation. If it comes with the [Page 100] thick and tough
humour, use Pills of cochia or Hiera, then drop in oil of bitter Almons. Rue or castor, with a little honey & Vinegar, also a toast very
hott with the Spirit of wine, or strong water sprinkled on it, apply'd
to the Ear is good. Sneezing powder is good in this case, neither
should clysters be omitted. Note that the former Medicines should
be applyed in the morning & before supper. If in fevers there happens this sounding in the ears, let it alone till the fever be ended.
If it continue after, use infusion of wormwood with water & Vinegar.

Pains of Ears

Sometimes the ear is grieviously pained, in other cases besides
the fever, by reason of could & other distempers. Rx. oyl of sweet
Almonds or lilly, or roses with brest milk, or bloody *water*, the drops

58. The tonsils were sometimes known as the almonds of the ears. "Almons
down" suggests that the remedy that follows was used to reduce swelling of the
tonsils.

from roasted beef, or apply green tobaccco leaves, moistned with water of Rue. If the paines be vehement, drop in juice of Purslain, lettice or henbane. If other things help not, give 3 grains of Laud. opiatum. [Page 101]

Eyes to cure

To draw out *things fallen into the* Eys: Pull the upper *lid below* the nether *and then throw the eye's lid off* etc. *as before. Or blow* [the nose]. *Or water or honeyed water into the* eys; a little milk or new milk. If lime *hath fallen into the* Ey *drop in the white of an egg. Also* sneezing *is good and sniffing, blowing of the nose.*

Ophthalmia or Inflammation of the Eyes

This Dissease is to be cured according to the severall causes, which are either inward or outward as Blood, choler abounding, outward *as small proud tumors.* Signs are rednes, heat, paine in the Eyes, teares, much filth coming *from eyes.* When this dissease comes from outward causes, they being removed, the cause ceaseth. If it comes from inward causes usually cupping, blood letting, purging cholerick humours with Rubarb or Syr. of roses solution. Or Syr. of Violets or Pil. lucis may be given many times. Sometimes the strait veine in the forehead may be opened. Washing the hands & feet before meals in cold water. Blisters behind the ears. A seton in the neck kept open many days. Mastichatorys are good to avoid humours out of the mouth.

TOPICK MEDICINES

Green leaves of the vine, bruised & applyed to the forehead, or leaves of the bramble bush, or purslane. Also bole Armoniack & sanguis draconis mixed with the white of egge, & Vinegar wherein red roses, red Saunders & frankincense have been boyled. Or take bole Armoniack, drag[on's] blood, mastick, roses, mixed with white of an egge, rose water and Vinegar, applyed to the temples & forehead. Or the juice of plantain with the white of an egge, but these must not be used if rumes (rheums) be great without purging, especially when we use restringents. Or take Sief album, sincopis, dissolve it in woman's milk and rose water or whites of egges with brest [Page 102] milk & plantain juice. Or with rose water dropd into the eye, Or take Vitriol alba & tutty prep of each 1 dram; dissolve therein rose water and drop the water into the Eye. Or white Vitriol dissolved in common water alone. The juice of Maywood *taken* first or last for 3 or 4 dayes together cures this malady. In the declining of the dissease, Sarcocolla dissolved in rose water or fennel water.

For a Pin and Web in the Eye or Unguis Oculi

Rx. Egge shells steeped in sharp Vinegar 6 hours. Then dry the Egge shells & make a powder of them, and blow it through a quill into the eyes. It cures this dissease without paine. Or take whites of egges that are hard sodden & rose water & a little white Vitriol & sugar candy; mix the things together with white of the egg cleft and clap both pieces together and squese it hot into the rose water, before the white of the egg be cold. Keep it in a glass, & so wash the eye with it 3 hours a day. Or take brest milk and honey, of each equal parts; add a little saffron & boyl them together & drop a little into the eye. Or Take Sumach & mix Gumm Arabic & Sarcocol (la) with it; put it into the Eye. Or take thin brass and steep it in urine 4 or 5 days, dryed & poudered. [Page 103] [One line illegible]. Steep the pith of young Sassafras in Spring water & wash in the eys often. Probat. est.

For the Dissease Albugo in the white of the Eye

This Dissease is a white spott in the white of the Eye, causing the Eye to see things as it *were* through a Cloud or smoke. To help the eye in young bodys, for in the aged this be hardly cured, Take the Vapour of the decoction of the herb Fenucrik, Mallows or Camomile, or of the chaff of barly, into the eye till the face be red with it. Then take ey-bright water & dissolve sugar Candy in it, & drop it into the ey. Stronger Medicines are made thus. Take the Gaul of a Cock or goose or eel or picke (pike) & mix it with fennel water or a little honey or pigeons dung. Also henbane juice dropped into the eye 15 dayes takes away this whitenes.

Film or Spot Roving in the Eye

Rx. Allom burnt in fine pouder, put into an egg well roasted. After the yolk is taken out while the white is very hott, clap the two peices together and squeeze it hard till the moisture comes out and wett a little further with the water and draw it through the eye two or 3 times a day. This is nothing so painfull as the oyl of Linnen raggs so used. [Page 104]

Wounds of the Eyes

Opening of a veine & purges of Rubarb are good in the beginning. Afterward let the white of an egg be mingled with Seif album that is to be had at the Apothecarys. Or take the white of an egg with 1 oz. or 2 oz. of rose water; ad allum and Saffron, of each 1 dram; mixe them and lay them in the wound, to hinder inflammation of the eye. Make a poultis of Mallalote and the heads of poppy, saffron & bread, and lay it on the ey lid, so that any filth may have free passage out of the eye. Afterwards take Gumm Arabic, 3 drams; Cream of Comfrey roots, 1¹/₂ oz.; small pouder of frankincense, washt Aloes, of each 1 scruple; mingle them for the healing the wound. After the 7th day, take Myrhhe, Sarcocolla, of each ¹/₂ dram; tutty prepared, 1 dram; honey or roses, q.s. F. ung. to heale up the wound. [Page 105]

For the blood shot of the Eyes

Rx. Decoction of Mellilote, Fenugreek & wash the eyes therewith. Or you may use infusion of fenugreek & myrrh. Also the blood of Pigeons & swallows are excellent in this case, and old blood shot mayst be holpen with wormwood or radish juice. Or Hysop bruised, tyed in a linnen cloth dipped in hot water & so applyed warm to the eye. Or take wormwood green bruised, mixed with breast milk & rose water.

A Suffusion of the Eye or Cattaract

A Cattaract is a gathering of some humour on the apple of the eye that hinders the sight wholly or in part. In the beginning of it motes or bodys like hairs or spiders Webbs appear before the eyes of the same colour that the humour is. Afterward the colour of the apple of the eye is blew or sea-coloured. Lastly the apple of the eye seems white & all light is gone. Then it is a cattaract & sometimes it posseseth one eye and sometimes both.

When it is curable, bleeding is good & purging with Hira (hiera) or Diacathamum (diacarthamum). Also let the patient take ivory with Treacle or Mithridate, 1 scruple or ½ dram mixed with Conserve of Anthos or betony. Also the decoction of Guaiacum, Sassafras or Sassaparilla with Celandine, Ey-bright, and Coriander seed prepared. Let the patient take it in the morning fasting. Also a seton kept open in the Neck 6 months is needfull. [Page 106] Blisters also behind the ears. Also Cauterys in the arms for revulsion. Also the Vapour of the decoction of ground Ivy with Eye bright & fennel seed is good. Also take the bladder of a fish emptyed & washt & filled with the decoction of fennel and apply this warm. Afterward it is good to drop into the eyes clarifyed honey, or honeyed *water, myrhh* & *dill* with a little sugar Candy. Also juice of rue, fennel or Calamint dropt into the eye is good. Or take the Gaul of a Cock mixed with Mouses blood & brest milk. If these things prevail not for the cure, you must proceed to manuell opperation & to pricking with a Needle. It must be done according to art & not be attempted by a young Chyrurgion.[59]

Things generally good for the Eyes

Pil. sine quibus, or Pil Lucis. Troches of Agric are good to purge the head & Comfort the Sight. Also roses, fennel, Vervaine, Soladine (celandine), rue, pimpernel, betony, oculus xti (Christi), ey bright, mellelote, washing hands often, especially before meales.[60]

Things hurtful for the Eyes

To eat Garlike, Onions, Leeks, mustard, much Lettice, to travail or study too suddenly after meals. Wine, hott liquours, looking upon snow, Drunkennes, gluttony, milk, cheese. Looking much upon white things. Much sleep after meat. Much bleeding. Coleworts, dust, fine smoak, reading small prints, reading immeadiately after supper, overmuch watching. [Page 107]

---

59. This procedure, known as couching for cataract, was a recognized specialty.
60. Palmer does not explain his reason for this sensible advice.

Succus Solani, the plant

stampt & apply'd to pained soar eyes *has done good to many*. For blood shott eyes, by hurt or otherwise, *for swollen* eys, *much pain* and soarness, Boyl rose leaves till they be soft. Wash oft with the water & at nights bind them warm upon the soar eyes. *This is used always with good* success. Much using of painfull medicines doth usually destroy the sight. Its a sure Rule for the eyes: use first that which is anodine, & after that abstersive.

Rx. Broom root steep'd in fair water. Take the blue scum that arises with a feather or ragg; drop it into the Ey. It will take of (off) the film & restore the sight. An indians medicine. Probatum est.

Face

To take away Pimples out of the Face. Rx. white wine Vinegar, brim stone, hony, pure wheat flour, F. ungt. & annoint with it going to bed. Use it 4 *or* 5 times. Or Rx. white Copperas, calcined & dissolved in water & warmed & wash with it. This is good for a high coloured face. Or take Nigella stampt & mixt with wheat flour, F. ungt. Annoint the face going to bed. [Page 108]

For a fry (inflamed) Face

Rx. Vine leaves, strawbery leaves, Camphire (camphor), Cream & distill them together & make a water to annoint the face. Or take Beer, Suet, and brimstone. F. Ungt. with white wine Vinegar, all boyld together, & annoynt the face with a little of it often. Also take every morning a cup of beer, wine or ale with english madder steeped in it. Or take Housleek, wild tansy, white wine, F. a lotion. Or wash with juice of Cucumber. Or Rx. Smiths water, Elder leaves, & bark, sage, allom, & make a decoction for to wash the face.

For a Leprous Face [61]

Rx. Litharge of Silver & brimstone of each alike. Seeth them in rose water & Vinegar, dip a Linnen cloth therein & lay to the face.

---

61. In this context leprous meant scaly.

Observation

In a Time of general Sicknes have a care of outward medicine to the breaking out & pimples of the face.[62] At other times if you use such medicines for beauty, look at the inward cause of such breakings out, & use suitable inward medicines according to the nature of the inward humour. [Page 109]

Falling Sicknes

This differs from Convulsion fitts because they are more constant & continuall. In the Epilepsy there is some distance between the fitts; a Convulsion of not a part only but the whole body and all the animal functions. There is a froth of the mouth, grinding of the teeth & rowling of the eyes.

The Remedy

In grown persons blood-letting, also frequent purging, either by Vomit or Seige as the cause may be. Decoctions of sage, Rue, Hyssop, rosemary, spirit of Vitriol, a few drops in spirit of wine, or a decoction of herbs, Oximel scilliticum, or Vinegar of squill, dayly taken every morning a spoonfull. Rx. Rue, Piony, Misselto of the Oak, Castor, Sage, Baccharum lauri, Cranum Human usto. Alike Treacle or Mithridate, Despumat. hony. F. Elect. The patient must purge every week. Pyrethrum mixed with hony & taken. Also decoctions of Guajacum, Sassafras & Sassaparilla taken some length of time, also lignum Coryli, laudatum valde. These things are commended, Pioni, Misselto of the oak, flowrs of the Nil tre (Nile tree), rue, Castor ungul. [Others, boar's bladder with urine dried in strings, dried frog's liver given fasting in wine, heart of wolf, boar's testes, horse's milk,][63] water of black cherys, *distilled water of swallows*. I cured (*thus* Dr. *Fuller*) by Gods leave a youth that [illegible] [Page 110] I gave 3 potions of working physick. It wrought much after I caused him to use a drink of seeds and opening herbs & castor

62. That is, consider whether the skin eruption is a symptom of some epidemic disease.
63. The passage in brackets is a translation of Palmer's Latin.

to use for some times & then let blood in the arm, & then his fitts left him.

Observation

I know one that had blisters, drawn & kept open in the Neck,[64] for a month together and all that time had no fitts of the falling sicknes & before had a great many, day after day, and for a long time. Oil of Vitriol is highly commended. Take a few drops in spirit of wine. [Page 111]

Flux. The bloody Flux

Spiders webb [illegible]. Stamped together, lay on the navil. Vid. Leesens[65] page 156.

Felons to cure

Rx. Rue, Soap, Fetherfew, salt, barrows greese, Verdigreese &c. Damp them & apply them.

Fevers

The names, kinds, causes, differences, so phillip Barrow & the genel (general) practise of physick, & the book called the breviari of health.[66] There be certain quartans, quotidians, simple & compound & several pestilential fevers. A Fever is an unnatural heat in the body, overspreading the whole body. It *is carried by divers kinds of* humours whether malignant or not. It is a companion of other distempers, as in children that have worms, convulsions, or breeding of teeth. In women its caused by obstructions.

The best Rule is consider the cause & help nature to expell her superfluities if she be not able or hindred. Take heed of deferring

64. The blisters, produced by cupping, were a form of counterirritation.
65. Not further identified.
66. See, respectively, Barrough's *The Method of Phisick*, page 215f. Wirtzung's *The General Practice of Physick, page 622f.* and Boorde's *The Breviary of Helthe, chapter 136.*

as many doe through carelesnes or other reasons. [Page 112] In time of general Sicknes if there be any symptoms of a fever invading the body and nothing forbid, take a Vomit presently. If need be after, a gentle sweating medicine.

Observation

In the year 1676 many fell sick and died in several Towns in N. England of a putrid Fever that proved very mortal. Divers by taking Vomits at the beginning did not die by it; others by taking a gentle sweat were soon well, but such persons as had not the use of such means, lay a long time altho they escaped with their lives. Many that bled much at the nose of their own accord did escape with their lives. Such as did take Vomits or purges or were let blood, if it were not in the beginning, lay a long time, or if they *took* sweating medicines. *Purges and sweating they took cured; and so shortened their lives.*[67]

Directions

As soon as paine in the head, bones or limbs, or sence (sense) of a chill coldnes be taken notice of, then presently either take a sweat or Vomit & keep house & warm two or 3 days, & if need be sweat a second time, if at night in a warm bed, if they can be carefully tended. I commend either Mithridate, [Page 113] Treacle, Carduus, Wormwood, salt of Wormwood, or Salt of Carduus &c., oyl of wormwood, peneroyal, Hysop & such like oyls. *It is vain to meddle with them if doubtless means do them work.*[68]

The most of them that had this Fever had a loosenes of body, and many a bloody flux. In these last cases some used purges of Aloes, others of Rubarb & divers times repeated, and some healing or comforting clysters. In time they were all profitable. Vid. Dr. Arnold's method at the latter end of the latine manuscript entitled Brevis physicae, Apendix. Salt of Tartar Dissolved in oyl of Tartar that is made by Deliquium. Add oyl or spirit of Vitriol, a few drops mixed together in a Vessel. A few drops of this for a fever in convenient liquor. [Page 114]

67. Did Palmer mean to say that these persons *lengthened* their lives?
68. "Vain" meant unwise: "doubtless," safe, without a doubt.

Fistula

It is a long and callous and hollow Ulcer, little painfull. Use Strong purges & Diet drinks to dry the body & corrupt humours, as by Guajacum. Then consider whether the Fistula be deep or shallow; if it be shallow, it must be laid open, without any cutting of great veines, or sinews. Then the cure will be easy, to eat out the callome, & to cure it as ordinary Ulcers. If it lyes deep & the orifice be narrow, it must be enlarged with a tent of Gentian or trochor (trocar) de minis, or a spurge thus prepared.

Rx. Cera, resinae, of each 1 oz.; sublimat, 1 dram. Liquescat. Postea adda sublimatum. Soak your spurge in the mixture, & presently pluck it out, & so put it into the orifice, then root out the callousnes thus. Fill the place with black hellebore or laserpitio succo. Or Rx. ungt. aegyptiacum, ½ oz.; sublimatum, ½ dram; Arsenici, 1 scruple; lixivii, ½ oz.; aq. ros., 2 oz.; Aqua plantag., 4 oz. Coquantur ad tertiam. Make hereof an injection. 2 or 3 days after the injection, close up the orifice with wax or bombast.

Sometimes this is done with handy operation as by a cautery or incision. If by incision, that incision is to be followed all along the hollow, to the very bottom of the fistulo. After you may take out the callus with your fingers or Instruments so that the quick and perfect flesh may everywhere appear. Incision and cautery is thus to be done together. If nerves and Arterys forbid not, first try with your probe which way the hollow runs and so follow the Probe with your incision knife. If there be many turnings, follow them in like sort with your Probe and Knife. Now when you are come to the end of your fistulo, fill up all the ulcer with [Page 115] tents & lints dipped in the white of an egge that the lips of it may be kept asunder. The day following burn the place with a hot iron, or Caustic [that is, with powder of asphodel or arsenic or mercury].[69] If the fistulo lye deep, you must not use incision but follow the former course, to take away the callum by injections of causticks. But after the fistulo hath been burned, the day following use oyl mixed with the yolk of an egge. When the

69. The passage in brackets is a translation of Palmer's Latin.

callus is gone, molify the ulcer with aqua mulsa. Where the fistulo is pure, use incarnatives.

Rx. Aqua vitae, 2 oz.; Vini malvatici, 1 oz.; mel rosati, ½ dram; Myrrhe, Sarcocolla, Aloes, of each, 1½ oz. Misceantur et coquantur. Hereof inject with a syringe for the whole cure of a fistelo. The easiest way is to make a broth of red colewort leaves & to give those oft to the patient, 3 times a day. If the part be not grown with callous flesh, it may be profit[able] by keeping the body soluble.

Observation

Where the bone is foule, it will never heale untill the scales do come off & that in length of time. By the use of good medicine, nature will generate good flesh that will grow to the bone & so thrust of the scale or scales. Before it be affected, it may be a year or two. The Tincture of Mars is one of the best Medicines for this use. See the preparation in the latter part of the book, Pag: 233. [Page 116]

The Falling of the Fundament

This is to be put up with the hand, the Patient lying on his belly. If it be swollen, bath it with the decoction of mallows, Camomile flours, Linseed, Fenugreek, butter & oyl Pills, decoction of red roses, plantain, balust, shepheards pouch, shumach, frankencense, or some of these made in water or red wine. Afterward the part is to be annointed with oyl of roses, or Myrtles, & the powder of Frankincense, mastick, & sanguis Draconis, galls, sumach sprinkled on. Then proceed according to the several Causes. If binding be the Cause, use soluble things. If sharpnes of humours be the cause, as in the bloody flux & tenasmus, the sharpnes of the humour must be tempered; if the membranes be loosned, the rupture must be closed, as in rupture. If there be a resolution of the part as in the Palsy, annoynt the part with oyl of bayes, Castor &c.

Observations

This Dissease is frequent in many children because of the moisture & sharpnes of humours flowing that way. [Page 117]

Gout

This Dissease pains the joints. It hath diverse differences, the knot gout counted incurable, nor that which is hereditary. Open a veine called Sciatica on the outside of the ankle *or rather* foot *below the* ancle. Cupping and Leeches, then Elect. Caricostinum is to be used. Use Vomits, Pil. Foetida, Hermodact. or Pil. Arthriti, decoctions of Guajacum, Sassafras, Sassaparilla. Also Fontinals & Setons are good. Also Acetum Nilliticum dayly taken cures all paines of the joynts. Also distilled water of broomflowers helps. Ould cheese plaisterwise apply'd helps much; some use green cheese.

To ease the Paine

Take Mallows leaves & roots, boyld in wine Vinegar till the third part be consumed. Mix some rye & bran and make a Poultis. Apply it warm. The water of Spawn of Froggs helps. Vid. J. Cooks works.

Also decoction of Parietory to bath withall. If these prevail not, use Henbane leaves, Night-shade berrys boyld soft, and barly meale, oyl of roses for a plaister. Or take barly meale, crums of wheat bread, milk; boyl it till it be thick. Add oyl of roses, yolks of eggs, Opium 3 drams. Or make a plaister with figgs and mustard seed, the seeds being first bray'd & after beaten together with figgs.

To draw out the Humour

Rx. Gum. Carann., 1½ oz.; Taecamahac, 2 drams; oxycrocei, 11 oz.; Cera alb., ½ dram or q.s.; pulv. consolid. majoris, 2 drams; cum ol. Chamomel. F. Empl. Also bathing the Feet with beif broth and Cabbage Leaves.

Or Rx. gum mastic [illegible],[70] [Page 118] [1 oz.; black pine pitch, 2 oz.; [illegible], 1 dram; fat of an old rooster, powder of Hermaodactyles compound, native sulphur, 2 oz. Make a plaster. Renew it in 30 days. Ammonia dissolved in vinegar is useful for dissolving tophi.

Or Rx. Old and sharp cheese, 5 oz., dipped in salt pork. Make a plaster.

70. The following passage in brackets is a translation.

Or Rx. tobacco juice, 3 oz.; candied citron, 2 oz.; pine rosin, 1½ oz.; terebinth, 1 oz.; camomile oil, as necessary. Make an ointment.]

For the Windy Gout, a great secret

Make a Curd with milk and wine Vinegar. Add to it a handful of black powder of white ashe wood, that is, it that beareth Keys. It may be on 12 or 24 hours. If it be in the left knee, bind the right arm about the elbow, & so the contrary part.[71] Its said it will do without binding & that the powder is the cheif. Anoynt with rum, Cream & sallade oyl, boyled to an oyl. [Page 119]

Gangreene

A Gangreen and Sephalus are [to be] distinguished, the first [being] the beginning of the latter. It tends to mortification of the part. It may be without any humour at all, so that the Gangreen is an imperfect Mortification, & if it be not speedily holpen, the member quite dies & looseth all sence and motion, & when it is come to that, it is called a Saphellus, and that takes not only the softer parts as flesh & Arterys & Nerves as a Gangreen only doth, but it is in the very bones and hardest parts. The cause of both maladys is the destruction of Natural heat either by too much cold, or some venomous quality, or by transpiration hindred, or by vehement outward heat, or by want of nourishment.

Signs of a Gangreen

The Colour of the flesh is changed, and it grows blackish and blew, & the pulse, sence & motion are diminished & heat that do encrease still more and more. When there is a perfect mortification, then the life, sence, and motion is quite lost in the part and though it be cutt or burned, it feeleth no paine. The flesh is cold; to sence, soft & black and stinking.

71. Obviously a charm.

The Cure of a Gangreen that Comes by Cold and Freezing[72]

When this Gangreen comes first, the part is red and the paine vehement and burning & then the frozen parts must not come near the fire, for then the parts do presently die. But the patient must be kept far from the fire. Yea, it is best to rubb the frozen part with snow or Ice or to hould it in the water till it should [Page 120] recover heat again. Then it is good to give the patient a draught of wine with Treacle or strong beer with Cinnamon, Cloves or Ginger, and so to cast him into a sweat in his bed, well warmed. Then when the paine is mitigated, it is good to cherish the parts with warm milk wherein bay berys, rosemary, Camomile & sage have been boyled. Afterwards boyled turneps apply'd for a poultis, will recover the parts wonderfully. Or oyl of turpentine. But if the Gangreen be present & the part mortify'd in pt. (part), then the part must be scarrifyed & fermented with the decoction of scabious, scordium, or Lond. Treacle & mithridate.

The Cure of a Gangreen that Comes from a Conflux of Venomous Humours

In this the Diet must be cooling & drying and meats must be seasoned with Citrons & Lemons and Pomgranates, and the patient must be purged and blooded. Cordials must be given dayly of Card. ben., scabious, borage, with Treacle and Mithridate & Bole Armoniak & Terra sigillata in a draught of ale M. & E. that if it may be, the venemous matter may be sweated out. And when the Venemous matter is within the body, no defensives may be used but only the swollen parts must be scarifyed & cupped or Leeches be apply'd to them, & the pt. must be often bathed with warm water, rue, dictamnus, Angelica, especially Scordium.

Lotion to make to syringe a foul running sore. Rx. A quart of rum, myrhh, Aloes, of each 1 oz. Steep them in the rum ready to boyl [illegible]. [Page 121]

72. Frostbite.

The Gangreen that comes by the biting of Serpents and Venemous Creatures

In this case the part affected must immediately be cut or scarified, and then such medicine must be applyed to the incision as may draw out the poison, as Pigeons dung, onions or garlick roasted in embers, mixed with Treacle or Mithridate. Lastly when the Venome is driven forth, the incision may be cured with the juice of Parsly or hony of roses.

The Gangreen that comes by Inflammation or Abundance of Blood

In this case the diet must be sparing and cooling & there must be purging of the whole body, and blood-letting, & defensives must be applyed about the part & the heart must be defended with Cordials of the decoction of Carduus and Mithridate & bole Armoniack being added thereto. The parts affected must be scarifyed, and washed with salt water or lye in which Aloes is dissolved and after the part is washed, apply ungt. Aegyptiacum & some times when there is a great flux of blood actual Cauterys with hot Irons is to be used. After Searing use Succum Porri or Sal cum porro that dry and resist putrifaction, the ordinary defensives in this case, i.e., argila cum aceto, clay mixed with Vinegar. Or Rx. juice of Plantain & semper vivum, or quinces, or the decoction of sumach, roses, plantain, adding bole Armoniack, Sanguis draconis & terra sigillata thereto with a little Vinegar of roses. Or take the powders only [Page 122] with rose water and Oxycratum (*it is vinegar and water*) and of the white of an egg. When a Crust or eskar is made with burning, pare it away with a knife. The rest of the cure is to be performed as in the cure of common ulcers.

The Gangreen from defect of Nourishment

In this case hott and moist food & such as begetts good blood & are easy of digestion. Anoynt the body outward with oyl of sweet Almonds, or other sweet oyl. All drying things are to be avoided. The nourishment is by means to be drawn to the decayed part or [part that is] beginning to be mortifyed. Therefore here is no use of defensives, because they hinder the spirits & blood from the mortifyed part. [73] The part affected is to be annoynted with oyl of earth-worms, or the juice of earth worms, first washed in water and then in wine & so put into a Vessel wherein is much oyl of sweet Almonds and so melted over a gentle fire and also Cupping glasses are to be applyed to the grieved part. Also salt water sod with Scordium or myrrhe are good, or tar with meale of Lupines. Scordium or Myrrh are good to be apply'd to the part grieved. If the Gangreen is begun, then the part is to be scarifyed and Aegyptiacum apply'd to the part scarifyed.

The total Mortification after a Gangreen and the Cure

When any part is quite mortifyed, it must be immediately cutt & if it be in such a place that the part cannot be cutt off the case is [Page 123] desperate. For the feet, Toes, fingers, privy members may be adventured to be cut off, but if it be in the brest or belly it may not be attempted.

When Incision or Amputation is to be used, the mortifyed part a fingers bredth from the same part is to be launched to the bone, & so the bone to be sawed off, and the rest of the flesh corrupted is to be burned with actual Cautery &c. Or also when the mortification is vehement, & creeping fast, the amputation is to be made in the sound [flesh] with searing up the Veins to prevent a great flux of blood. In the latter case, which is to be thought the best way of cure, the paine may be mitigated with strait binding of the part & the sharpnes of the incision. [The] knife will soon dispatch it. Besides, it is better to stop the flux of blood with strait binding after ampu-tation than is to do it by Cautery, which bring many disconveniences and greater paines. Be wary in these *cases*, ex gr, [I] *have seen the lurkings of these things occurring often.* [74]

Observation

I once saw a Child (*thus* Dr. *Fuller*) that had a *swelling* sudden and painfull, being an ulcer and the beginning of a Gangreen, whose

---

73. Since the gangrene arises from lack of nourishment, therapy is recommended that will draw nourishment into the affected area. Defensives, q.v., are contraindicated.
74. Be wary of subtle changes.

Father tould me (he being the principle Chirurgion in the Cure) [that] blackish blew spots arose in the part and it *was* stopt from encreasing by applying a plaister about the part of Ruffi's pills (pilulae Rufi) made of Myrrh, aloes & safron. Vid. James Cook 'Of Gangreen.'

To stop a Gangreen Scarrifie every where where it appears & put in pouder of bay salt & white copperas, of each equal parts. If the water will issue out in a hard [illegible]. [Page 124]

Gonorrea Running of the Reines[75]

This disease cometh from the weakness of the retentive Faculty in the Seminal Vessels. It comes often to those that live a single life & are grown to years. In the former case commonly drying and astringent things profit, as red roses, Coral, Sumach, Terra sigillata, hartshorn burnt, flours of Pomegranates. Of *these* together or some of them, F. potion.

Rx. ol. rosarum, mastic, myrtels, pomegran. flours, wax. F. ungt. pro renibus. But if the disease be joyned with coldnes, medicines may be prepared of Mastic, Frankencense, mints, Spik[enard]. Let the secret parts be bathed with oyl of mints, mastick & wormwood. Especially in this case, binding and artificial baths are good. If the Semen be hott & sharp, cooling medicines must be used.

Rx. Four great cooling Seeds, 3 drams; Purslain, Lettuce, of each 1 dram; Flours of roses, 1 1/2 drams; water Lillies, 1/2 dram; Gum Tragacanth, 1/2 dram. F. a powder. If the Semen be thin and watry, use drying & corroborating medic[ines] as mints, Roman wormwood, 1 minim; Sem. agnus castus & leaves of Myrrh, flowers of red rose, 2 drams, boyld in red *wine* and sweetned with sugar. For the diet, rice sod in milk is the best. If the sem[en] be corrupt and virulent, abstain from astringent medicines, but yet you must use drying medicines as Mithridate especially. And Virulent humours are to be purged out with decoction of Guajacum, [Page 125] sassafras, and Sassaparilla, also lye made with the stalks of beans brought into ashes, 4 oz., being given every day.

75. It was erroneously believed that the gonorrheal discharge was from the kidneys.

Observations

Eat frequently Indian beans with fleet milk and samp and parsneps water wherein Iron hath been quenched; flowers, leaves, and roots of water lillys; pills made of Turpentine & Nutmeg, or Enula Roots. [Page 126]

Head Ach

Consider the divers causes, whether it come from outward accidents or from within and if from within, it come from the distemper of head it self or by the consent of parts. [If] it comes from any outward cause, it will appear by the relation (account) of the sick [person]. If it come from the consent of other parts, it is by fitts. The Urine commonly sheweth the Dissease, as in fevers it is commonly troubled like a beasts urine. They have always the head ach. Also if urines which in the Dissease are made clear are not easily troubled, it is a signe of the head ach. Also small bubles spread over the Crown of the water is a signe of the head ach, and the paine is sharp when the bubles are yellow, milder if they be white, long if they continue long. When the paine is great, the juice of the Muscilage of Mallows with oyl of roses and brest milk applyed easeth the paine. So [does] the decoction of Camomile flowrs or wheat bread, moistned with warm milk. And if these suffice not but paine and head ach & watching continues, we must use Narcotiques and such as cause sleep, as Lettice, Nymphea, Solanum, Mandragora, Opium, Philonium Rom[anum], Requies Nicolai, Pil. de Cynoglossa, 1 to 2 scruples. Or Laudan. opiatum, 2 or 3 grains. When the Head ach is caused by the distemper of the head we must see whether it come by blood or phlegm, Choler or Melancholy, & accordingly direct the cure.

For the purging of each humour, in a cold distemper use this Epithime. Rx. Pulv. Zeadoric, 1 dram; aqua betonica, verbane Sambuci, of each 1 oz. In all sorts of head ach the distilled water of Vervain is a great secret, both to apply it outwardly to the head and to [illegible] [Page 127] 4 or 5 oz. with spirit of salt, 3 Gut. (*guttae*) the [illegible] and laying about the neck is admirable or to lay the herb to the Crown. If *the head ach come then let mild heat as the sun or slight wind. Then apply to the head things that are a little cold, as cold water, etc. The head ache if it come by nose bleed or cancer, early death but in* [skull] fracture *there is* blood letting and clysters. Shave the head & annoynt with oyl of Roses & myrtles mixed therewith. In like manner the Hemicrane or Cephalea, or the ach of one side of the head and cured with opening of a Vein in the forehead or Nostrils. Also the decoction of Guajacum, sassafras & sassaparilla are precious in this case. [Page 128]

Hicket or Singultus

The Common Hicket is easily holpen. Take thy fingers ends and stop both thy ears very hard, & this malady will soon be gone. Also drink a very long draught of drinking while together.[76] This will stop it.

There is a Hickup in acute Fevers that is a sad symptome & dangerous, and this is hard to cure. Rx. Bole Armoniack with borage, or bugloss water, or purslain water, or wine of Pomegranate, Conserve of Roses, Vitriolate. If this help not, give Laud. opiat., 3 grains, or Philon. Roman. or Treacle, and apply to the Stomach outwardly a Cupping glass with much flame. Also annoint the stom[ach] with oyl of wormwood. Or Lillys or Dill is good. A *fomentary but this is good:* oyl of Annis[ee]d oft taken. [Page 129]

Heart Distemper

First, the most common distemper of the heart is by heat, for all Fevers do come from thence. The distemper is known thus. 1. The breathing is quick & frequent. 2. Pulse great and frequent, quiet if the strength continues. 3. Pronenes to anger. 4. The whole body is hot especially lips, tongue, pallat & breath.

Medicines that cool the heart, Sorrel, Viola, flours of roses, borage, buglos, juice of Citrons, Lemons, Pomegranates, cherrys, fruit of ribs & barberys, heartshorn, Terra sigillata, bole Armoniack, Coral,

---

76. That is, swallowing steadily without interruption.

Pearl, waters of roses, Violets, Nymphea, *sorrel, borage, bugloss,*[77] strawberys, syrup. Acet. of Citri, Diamarg[ariton] frig., Conserves of the said hearbs before named.

There may be outwardly applyed Epithimes of rose *water* or Nymphea, Vinegar or roses, saunders, pearl, Coral, Camphir, bags of the hearbs, flours, or leaves of the fore named in a scarlet bagg. This must be apply'ed to the region of the heart, inside the left pap. Or we may use oyls or oyntments of the same. Besides all of this if blood abounds, a vein is to be opened and the body is to be purged with Rubharb, syr. of roses solutive, syr. of Violets, pulp of tamarinds, manna, Triphora, Bresica, &c.

Cold distemper of Heart

This Distemper is known by the weaknes, slowing & thinnes of pulse & such a breath also. The air breathed out appears cold, and sometimes the whole body is cold.

Medicines that heat the heart: Balm, rosemary, Card. Bened., Calamint, Angelica, Rosemary flowers, Lavender, Lilly of the Vallys, Citron seeds, grains of Alchornes, Lignum aloes, Cinnamon, [Page 130] Cloves, Zeadeary, Mace, Nutmegs, Amber, Musk, of these there be divers compositions, waters & spirits, Conserves, syrups, and preserves, oyls & species, besides confection of Alkermes, Treacle & mithridate, all sorts of aqua vitae, Electuarys.

Rx. Conserve Borag. Buglos, Anthos tunicis, of each 1 oz.; ros[e] ½ oz.; Cortex Citri condit., 6 drams; Nux Moschat. condit., 1 dram; pulv. Caryophill, ½ scruple; cum Syr. tunicis. F. Elect.

Moist Distemper of Heart

It may be known by the causes that went before, and by the effects, the softnes of the Puls and moistnes of the whole body.

Drying Medicines are good, as Pearls, Coral, hartshorn, bone of harts, bole Armoniack, Terra Sigellata, precious stones. The Diet must be drying.

---

77. It is not clear why Palmer repeats these names in shorthand after having just listed them.

Dry Distemper of Heart

This is known by precedent causes, as Cares, Sorrows, watching, hot & dry air, drinking much wine, fevers, especially the Hectick. The whole body pines and is dryed. The Puls is hard. It is cured with moistening medicines, as Borage, Buglos, Violets, the greater cooling seeds, raisins & almons. Also a warm bath of sweet water, with Mallows & Fenugreek sod therein. Also fomentations be made hereof. After the brest should be annoynted with oyl of [Page 131] sweet Almonds or Violets. The Diet must be moistning, such as in a Hectick Fever.

Palpitation or Passion or Beating of the Heart

There is somehow a continuall beating and troubling at the heart that comes by hurtfull vapours [that] the heart labours to drive away. The Malady is known by laying the hand upon the heart. Sometimes the patient cannot endure his hand to be taken away from it.

For the cure, if blood abound open a vein. The Hemorrhoids [vein][78] is a great help in this disease. Gentle purges, oft repeated. Oyl of Citrons is a special help, given with some conserves to rid away vapours. Also Raponticum 2 scruples, given in wine. Or take conserve [of] Batones, Rosemary flowrs, buglos, of each 1 oz.; Cortex citri Condit, red condit, Scorzonera, of each ½ oz.; Species Diamoses dulcis, [Species] Diambre, of each 1 dram; Confect. Alchorines, 1 dram; cum Syr. tunicis. F. Elect.

Rx. Conserve borag, tunicis, of each 1 oz.; Confect. Alchorin., Theriaca, of each 1 dram; Species Elect. de Gemmis, Aremat. rosat. letific. Galeni, of each 1 scruple. Cum Syr. Bugl. & de Cort. Citri. F. Elect.[79] [Also there may be applied externally bags with Melissa flowers, lavender, rosin, borage, bugloss or white wine & water of musk roses.]

If the troubling of the heart come of water contained in the pericardium, then use these Medicines. Rx. Confect. Alchor., Species Diambr., [Species] Daimosch., [Species] Aromat. Rosat., Theriac,

---

78. See n. 60.
79. The following passage in brackets is a translation of Palmer's Latin.

Mithrid[ate] & the infusion of Guaiacum, sassafras, saffaren (saffron) [Page 132] cum corticibus Citri, & without (externally) its good to apply new hot bread.

If this dissease is by the consent of other parts, as by the Spleen &c, there must be purging and blood letting & medicines for the Spleen and Hypochondres.[80] Also Cauterys & Vesicatorys in the arms & legs is good, only in this case Cantharides may not be used but rather Crow-foot, also Bezoar, perle, precious stones & treacle.

OBSERVATION

Some commend amber-greise, 3 grains taken at a time for 5 times following being mixt with Castor. Some have been cured with Castor only, some with Bezoar. Others have died within a few hours after Bez[oar was] taken.[81] [Page 133]

Hemorrhoids or Piles

This Dissease is taken for (related to) that flux of blood that comes from the Veines of the Fundament. Sometimes they do swell and are inflamed and do put men to paine. Sometimes they doe pour forth blood; but commonly they are distinguished by secret and blind Hemorrhoids which are within the body. Sometimes they are open and without the fundament to be seen. The Hemorrhoids flowing moderately and in convenient time do preserve a man from many Disseases, & [are] by no means to be stayed (coagulated). *Thus if they be stayed and do flow,* immediately they cause dropsy, consumption, blindnes, madnes. When the Piles do flow immoderately, they must be stayed with a Pledget of hares down, dipped in this ensuing medicine.

Rx. Pulv. Aloe, Frankincense, balust, Sang. Dracon., of each ½ oz. Let them be incorporated with the white of an egg & so applyed.

---

80. Some parts of the body were thought to have a "sympathy," or relation, with other parts. In this case, medicine for the spleen would be expected to benefit the heart.

81. Note the author's caution regarding the use of bezoar, a remedy of dubious reputation, although Culpeper praises it as a cordial (*Pharmacopeia*, p. 52).

It is good if the strength of the patient will suffer so to open a veine in the arm or fist to ease the Paine.

Rx. Fresh butter, oyl of roses, of each 1 oz.; Cerusa, *white lead*, washed, 1 oz. Grind them in a leaden mortar for an unguent. Or if the paine be vehement, take the yolk of an egg, oyle of roses, Juice of poppy or henbane. If this do not prevail, ad of opium, 1 scruple. Also mullein is good being *taken* inward in broth or milk boyled. Also fresh Treacle, Philonium Romanum, or Laud. opiatum may be given inwardly. When the Hemorrhoids are swollen without bleeding they must be opened [illegible]. [Page 134]

Roast an Onion in the embers with an Ox Gaul (oak's gall) and apply this. Also Aloes taken inwardly helps forward (advance) the Hemrhoids. Also strong wine being drunk. Also the juice apply'd to the swollen Hemorrhoids do open them. If need be horse Leeches apply'd to the fundament. When they are full & fallen off, the Pile must bleed as long as they will. The best is to sitt over warm water. [Page135]

Hernia or a Rupture

Sometimes there is a swelling of the Groins or Cods by reason of falling down the Gutts and sometimes by the falling of the Call (caul). Sometimes by both mixed together. Sometimes it proceeds from a waterish humour, sometimes from wind, sometimes a fleshy excrescence of growth about the testicle.

The Cure of a true Rupture or Hernia

This is that which is commonly a Rupture when the Gutts or Call doth fall down into the Groine or Cods. Causes are Violent Motions, Stroaks, falls, Vomitings, Cough, leaping, rong (injury) by riding, lifting heavy burth[ens], viscid and windy meats. Such things may either relese or break the Peritoneum or that which is a thin & extended Membrane.

Signs the Peritoneum is broken

Are the suddaine increase of the humour and a sharp and cutting paine. When the Periton. is only relaxed, the humour groweth only

by little and that with small paines. Yet such paines return so often
as the humour is renued by the falling down of the Gutt or Caul. A
perfect (complete) and ould rupture by the breaking of the Peritoneum in men of full growth is seldom or never cured. But we must
note by great Ruptures of Peritoneum the Gutts may fall into the
Codd the bignes of a mans head without much paine or danger of
Life, because the Excrements as they may easily enter by reason of
the largenes of the place [illegible], so also they may readily [Page
136] returne.⁸²

CURE

First the patient shall be laid on his back either on a Table or bed,
so that his head shall be lower but his hinder parts higher. Then
shall he force with his hand by little and little and gently thrust the
gutts with his hand into the proper place, and then this fomentation
shall be applyed to the Groines.

Rx. Pomegranate pills, Cypris roots, galls, rock Allom, horse-tayl,
Sumach berrys, buglos in smiths water. [Take] of this infusion q.s.
Add meale of bean and barly, of each 1 oz.; powder of Aloes &
mastic, mirtles, sarcocolla, of each 1 oz.; bole armoniack, 2 oz. Of
these make a Cataplasm for the same purpose.

Rx. Contra Rupturam: also use this drink. Rx. Fearne that is
young, 5 or 6 handfulls; when it is a handfull or two high brew this
in 4 or 5 gallons of bear and let the beer be well boyled and let the
patient use this drink for 30 or 40 dayes. The cure consists in folded
clothes, Trusses, ligatures artificially made that the gutts may be
continued in this place. For the same purpose the patient must be
kept in a cradle or bed 30 or 40 dayes together & also must be kept
from crying or coughing.

Or Rx. Paper; steep it 3 dayes in water and apply it made in a ball
to the place, the gutts being first put up, for that remedy by 3 dayes'
adhesion will keep it from falling down. But this will be more effectual the paper being steeped in the former astringent smith's
water. Or beat a Load stone into fine powder and give it in [Page

82. That is, the canal through which the intestines have descended is large enough
that the passage of intestinal contents is not hindered.

137] pap, and annoint the groines with hony, and then strew it over with fine filings of Iron.[83] Let this Medicine be used for 10 or 12 dayes, the patient being well trussed up. Also red snails dryed in an Oven, in powder used to be given in pap or broth. Also Comfrey Roots, sanicle, Solomons Seale, thorowax, horse tailes, taken in infusion for 10 or 12 days, are very effectual.

Rx. Thorowax, Comfry, Mount royal, Solom[on's] Seale, roots of Polipody &c. F. Empl. Perfoliata is excellent in this case. [Page 138]

Hydroc[e]le

Thin & watery humour in the Cods, gathered by little and little. The Signs are an humour gathered by little, encreasing slowly, without much pain, heavy and almost a glassy clearnes, which you may perceive by holding a Candle on the other side. By pressing the Codd above, the water floweth down, and by pressing it below, it riseth upwards, but this can never be forced up into the belly, as the caul or gutt may, for often *times it is contained in a bag.*

The Cure must first be tryed with resolving, drying, and discussing medicines.

Rx. Cummin seed, 2 ½ oz.; bayberries, 2 oz.; salt, 1½oz.; brimstone, 1 dram. F. infusion in lye. To 3 parts conium.[84] Dip sponges in infusion; lay it to the Cod. After the fomentation, take bean flour, 3 oz.; linseed, fenugreek, powder of Camomile flours, Mollilot (melilot), of each 1 oz.; Cummin seed, ½ oz. Add oyl of Camomile and Rue. F. Empl.

Or take wax, 1 lb.; Terebin[th], 2½ oz.; Bedellium, Ammoniacum, of each 2 oz.; for a plaster. Or use ungt. Arippe & Arrogan. Also goat's dung with Sulphur apply'd.

If these means do not prevaile, the Cod must be opened below by incision & the bagg must be peirced without touching the testicle. [Page 139]

83. The iron fillings adhering to the lower abdomen and magnetically attracted by the loadstone in the stomach would be drawn up, reducing the rupture.
84. Palmer omitted something here.

The pnumatocle (pneumatocele) & Cure

That is a flatulent humour in the Cod generated by weaknes of heat in the part.[85] It is known by the roundnes, shining & prevelency. It is a swelling without heaviness. It is cured by prescribing a convenient diet, by the application of medicines that dissolve and diffuse flatulence, as seed of Annise, fennel, fenucreek, Agnus Castus, Rue, Organum.

Also Empl. Diacalcitheos. Dissolve in muscadine or other strong wine with oyl of bays. Also oyle of Rue, Cammomile, bay is good for an Ungt., or the plaster [of] bayberys. Abstain from windy meat.

Observation

[Illegible] *was a swelling in the* cod *of a sickly miller, a single man, a swelling as big as a g*[rown] *man's head, and by the nates, but keeping upon the back side* of the thighs close to the buttocks. The greatest *part of it was driven away,* drawing away at several times the greatest part of a pint of blood and water. [Page 140]

Herpes

Ring-worms or Tetters. It is a humour caused of choler. It is so called because of taking and spreading in the skin.[86]

For Cure, Medicines purging choler should be used & clysters are good.

For local medicines, Rx. Ceruss & Tutty prepared, 1 oz.; oyl of Roses and Capens (capon's) fatt, of each 2 oz.; the bark of pine burnt, ½ oz.; wax, q.s. F. ung.

Or Rx. juice of tobacco, 1 oz.; wax, ½ oz.; Resin pine, 1 oz.; turpentine, 1 oz.; ol. Myrrh, q.s.

85. The scrotum over the pneumatocele is relatively cool.

86. An interesting example of early dermatology. Palmer evidently considered ringworm and tetter to be synonymous with herpes. Dunglison (1868) equated herpes with tetter and regarded ringworm as another form of herpes. Now ringworm, herpes, and tetter are recognized as separate entities.

Or take cups of acorns, leaves of willows, leaves of brambles, lettice, Plantaine, houseleech (houseleek), Sempervivum. Boyl them in sharp wines. F. Cataplasm.
Or take ung. Diapomphol. Apply it.
Or Rx. burnt wool and pine bark burnt & washed fatt of a goat and wax. F. Emplastr.

Observation

Purging Diet drinks and salts of herbs to purge the humour out of the blood, taken for some time together, and the use of proper Diet to hinder such humours or expell them or change the nature of them. [Page 141]

Hydrocephalus

This humour groweth in the heads of Infants newly born. This humour is enclosed between the skull and the skin. The Tumour is soft & without paine, yeilding easily to the pressing of the fingers and sometimes the fore head huncheth out.
For the spreading of the watry humour, use a diet drink & let the child be kept soluble. Boyl Calamint, Peniroyal, sage, sawin, chamomile in Lees or sower wine & bath the head. Also Crowfoot to the neck causing blisters is a great Secrett. For this the infusion of Gaujacum is good [Page 142 is blank. Page 143]

Jaundice and the Cure

It is a Dissease that changeth the colour of the Skin; it is yellow or black. The yellow is caused by the obstruction or overflowing of the gaule.
Clysters & things purging choler are good to begin withall, as Rubarb Vomits are good. Also the opening roots are good in broth. Also Cream of Tartar washed with steeled wines is excellent taken divers days together. Also the infusion of prepared steele in *wine* drunk divers days.
Or take goose dung dissolved in white wine. Straine and drink it 2 hours before meat. Or take great earth worms. Wash them and

slice them & take scraped Ivory, English Saffron in powder. Mix
these together in white wine & let the patient drink a good draught
M & E. Or use infusion or barbery bark.

Or Rx. Turmerick, saffron, Myrhh & mix them. F. a powder; give
½ oz. at a time. Nep given in wine 3 nights together. Also Sassafras
roots or the juice. Very precious.

Black Jaundize

Rx. prepared steele, 2 oz.; passul. minor, 1½ oz.; infuse it 3 days
in aqu. cuscute et sucueri (succory) in a vessel close stopt with water.
Let it be seperate. Add root of sorrel, Polypody roots & bark of
Capers, Ceterach, madder, cuscuta, seed or agri[mo]ny, genistre
(genista). Boyl *it; in the course of* boyling ad Sena, 1 oz. *Take it off
and* add Syr. Scolopend., bizant. simpl., of each 1 oz.; sachar., q.s.
F. Syr.

Thus in like manner the melancholy is to be purged away. Use
infusion of camomile flours, Scordium, fennel root, red peas.

Also take a fish called a tench, cut through the back, and apply it
to the navel or to the Soals of the feet.[87]

Also *take a rooted harefoot.*[88] *Put the* white of geese dung with it in
wine or beer, first & last, warm. [Page 144]

Rx. Sheeps-dung steept in Milk 3 mornings. Probat. est. [Page
145]

Impostumes in the Body

Take the roots of Lillys and of flour de luce and stamp them
together. Add to them of hony a quart and boyl them all together
with wine and ale and being well sod, straine out the liquor & let
the patient drink first and last 2 or 3 spoon fulls at a time.

---

87. Another example of the theory of animal transference. The body of the fish,
split open, was expected to draw out the disease through the navel, site of a former
opening of the body, or down and out through the soles of the feet.

88. It is not clear whether Palmer means the animal foot or *Trifolium felinum*,
known as haresfoot.

Or take Centaury, rosemary, wormwood and horehound, and make them in a Syr. with white wine, and let the sick drink thereof, and it will breake the impostume but use it still. [Page 146]

Itch of Scab

There be 2 special kinds of the Itch. One, dry, is a dry scurf upon the body, the other moist & breaking out in watry wheals and scabs.

First use preparations to purge, Chicory, maiden hair. Then purge with rubarb & agarick & senna. Take whey of Goats milk and clarify it with leaves of cicory, borage, endive, fumitory, leaves & tops of each, 1 oz.; one root of fennel & cicory bruised; raisins, 1 oz.; and let them be sod in the whey, and drink fasting for 7 or 8 days seq.

Also Rx. senna, 1 minim, in a pott close stopt. Sod in whey with anniseed. Take it fasting, and take thin broth after it. When you have sufficient purged, procure sweat with infusion of Sarsaparilla, adding water or Syr. of fumitory.

Also baths of whey are good. Also make liniments of Hellebore and roots of flourdeluce boiled in Vinegar, adding hogs fat or fresh butter, also juice of sorrel.

Or Rx. litharge washed in Vinegar, roots of lillys, of each 2 drams; turpentine, 1 dram; ceruss, q.s.; juice of sharp pointed dock or senna, 1 oz.; common salt & oyl, q.s. F. ung.

Or take roots of enula, sharp pointed dock, of each 2 oz.; boyled in Vinagar and searse them. Ad turpent[ine], 2 oz.; ceruss, 1 oz.; 2 yolks of eggs; Allum, 2 drams; wine vinegar, a little. F. ung.

Or take 2 or 3 lemons & wring out the juice. Take the like quantity of oyl of roses & beat them well together & so annoint the part.

Likewise oyl of Myrhh healeth all manner of Itch or scabs and pimples, chaps & burning.

Or Rx. Brimstone, burnt Allom, ginger, of each ½ oz., and beat them very small and boyl them in bears greese, and so annoint the Itch.

Or Take Gun-powder with goose greese or hogs fatt, or you may add litharge and sulph[ur] with it. Or merc[ury] sublimate, mixed oyls or ung[uent] after the body [is] purged well.

Or quick silver killed with juice of lemmons, hog fatt, oyl of baye. [Page 147] beaten in a stone mortar, is a sure remedy, the body purged and sweated before. It *will be dangerous to use; it harms.*[89]

Or use a quick silver girdle made on this wise. Take Quick-Silver and minte (alter) it with fasting spittle, a great quantity, and being both mixed together in a bottle, they must be shaked together a whole day. And then dip a list (strip) of white English Cotton in it, and then let the list hang up in a chimney a day or two, and then wear the list upon the skin under the shirt a long time. This prevents lice. See the direction in some other [of] my writings about *making the* girdle. [Page 148 is blank. Page 149]

Kidnys, their Dissease and Cure

The Distemper of the Kidnys, hott and drye. [1.] There is heavines of the back, abundance of thin urine with fat swimming on the top, and often gravel in bottom. 2. Pronenes to lust, night pollution, & lustful desires. 3. Leannes of the body.

Cure of hott distemper is by cooling things; the dry distemper, by moistning things: distilled water of strawberrys, Violets, syr. of Violets, sorrel, syr. of Vitriol, mixed with cooling things.

Or greater cooling seeds, barly water, strawberry water, make an emulsion. Julep of roses or violets.

Outwardly, oyl of Nymph[aea], ung. Rosatum, Ceratum santalinum, vine-leaves, or lettice, or willows laid under the sheets.

A Plat of Lead to the Kidneys, not to the spine bone. A bath of sweet waters. Use barly cream. *Therefore use cooling seeds: rose, lettuce,* Cicory (chicory), endive, strawberys, *barley water,* small drink. If choler abound, a purge of cassia, electuarium psyllium, or of juice of roses.

Coldnes of the Kidnys

Urine little, thin, raw.[90] Little or no lust. If phlegm abound, urine thick and troubled. Thick and white threads appear therein.

89. A reference in shorthand to the toxicity of mercury.
90. Painful urination.

Use heating medicines: roots of fennel, Parsely, burnet, Ering
roots, Satyrium, sperage, betony, Agrimony, Calamint, mints, sage,
rosemary, lavender flours, spices. Annoint the reyns with oyl of nard,
Irees, mints, ung. martiatum. Purge with Cassia, turpentine, benedicta laxitiva.

Stone in the Kidneys

Signs: [1.] great paine in the Kidneys, sometimes in one, sometimes in the other. [2.] Stone falling in the uriterys (ureters), paines
more grevious & lower. 3. A bloody water. 4. Benummednes (numb-
ness) of thighs. 5. Sometimes vomiting & badnes of the stomach.
6. Fixedness & setledness of this paine, till gravel be voided.
[Page 150]
Vomiting is good once a month. If the cholick be joyned with it,
use gentle purges, Syr. ros. so., Cassia, manna, Rubarb, turpentine.

Rx. Hydromel, aqua Asparag., Syr. of Cicory with Rubarb tartari
Vitriol, 2 scruples, Misce for 4 days.

Turpentine in pills with powder of Liquorice and sugar.

If blood abound, open a veine in the Arme.

After those use saxifrage roots, burnt parsly, fennel, burdoch, radish, capers, betony, maidenhair, ground Ivy, broom flours, parsly
seed, Ivy berrys, red peas, bitter almonds, peach Kernels, berrys of
sweet brier, winter Cherys, amber, juice of Citrons and lemmons.

To prevent this dissease its good dayly to take turpentine as much
as a hasel nutt and swallow it every day with sugar, ground Ivy
however taken, also peach Kernels, strawberry water.

Rx. Purslaine water or juice, 1 dram; gum Arabick, 1 dram. Take
them half an hour before supper.

But if the stone be already generated, first blood must be let, and
a gentle purge given. After, diuretical things must be given & clysters.

A Purge. Rx. Cassia, 6 drams; Rhubarb, 2 scruples; Turbith, 1½
scruples; liquorice powder with sugar. F. Bolus.

A Clyster. Rx. rad. Althea, 1 oz.; Violets, mallows, brank-ursine,
parietory, of each 1 minim; summitatum Antho, ½ minim; flour
Chamomile, p.i.; sem. Fenucreek coq. in aqua colat., 4 lb.; ol. Viol,
2 oz.; cassia, 1 oz. F. a clyster. Foveatur locus vesica with sweet

water warm taken or milk. The reynes annoynt with oyl of sweet almons, or oyl of white lillys, or fatt of Goose or fresh butter, ung. Dialthea or oyl of scorpions. Also a bath of warm water with mallows sodd in it to open the passages. Cupping Glass applyd to the back lower than paine till the stone come to the blather (bladder).

THINGS AGAINST THE STONE

[Sponge stone, crab eye, a little stone taken from the bladder of a boar or cow, the jaw of a pike, lithontriptic compound.][91]
Rx. Goat's blood prepared, Sea horse pizel, salt peter, of each.[92] F. pulv. Abstain from salt meats, cheese, shell fish, mutton, veale. Yolks of eggs be good.[93] [Page 151]

Loyns ulcerated or Kidneys

Flash paine in the loyns with heavines, yet the water is made freely. Some filthy matter is made with the urine, and sometimes blood and sometimes little pieces of flock. In a full body open a veine in the arm. Use Violets, mallows & Nymphea, the 4 greater could seeds. Use barly, liquorice, raisens; gentle purges are good. Syrup of Violets & roses, solutio Diacatholicon, the lenitive electuary, especially Turpentine with liquorice. Hony water is good for drink, and the infusion of barly, pease and maiden-hair.

Or Rx. roots of Comfrey, china sassafras, and liquorice; sod, dissolve in the Conserve of red roses. Also use infusion of Guajacum. [Page 152 is blank. Page 153]

Kings-Evil

Its called Struma or Scrophula, and it is an oedematus humour that ariseth in the brests or arm hole or groine, but chiefly in the

91. The passage in square brackets is a translation of Palmer's Latin.
92. The amount is omitted.
93. In this and the preceding prescription, note the inclusion of bladder calculi and sea horse pizzle, an application of the theory of *similia similibus curantur*.

neck.[94] It differs from other humours in the number, for usually there appears many of them nodes united together. Some of them are moveable; others, woven with the nerves, immovable. These are the worst.

The cure. Purge the body frequently. Purge phlegm and melancholly. Let the diet be slender and sparing. Rx. roots of philupendula, 2 minims; scrophularia, 3 minims; Tansy, 1 minim; red colewort, 1 minim; the infusion of these in white wine and honey till half be consumed & being strained, give the party every S[econd] day 2 oz. in the morning fasting. This will purge by urine.

Or Rx. a new sponge, raw and washed. Infuse it in beer q.s., and being well sod and boiled at M.E. let it be taken.[95]

Or Rx. the ashes of a sponge burnt long and black, peper, ginger, Cinnamon, galls of an Oak, roses, of each 1 oz.[96] Make a powder and let the patient drink of this oft, and sprinkle it on his meats. Topic medicines as Diachilon magn[um] or coucumer or Diapalm[a].

Or Rx. Goat's dung mixed with hony and vinegar, or Cow dung and vinegar. Or Rx. Bran meale & barly meale, 1½ oz.; Liquorice, 1 dram; pitch and white wax, goose fatt, child urine. F. Empl.

If the matter will not be resolved, you must ripen it with a plaister made of barley meale, pitch, olibanum, urine of a child. When it is fully suppurated, open it with an instrument. Then wash it oft with buttr, and if any yet remaine, apply ung. Agripp(e) & so heale the ulcer as other soares. [Page 154]

---

94. Scrofula is now known to be a tuberculous infection of the lymph glands of the neck. It was once believed that the disease could be cured by the touch of the monarch. In Palmer's day scrofula was confused with struma or goiter, a quite separate disease also characterized by swelling of the neck. Wirtzung stated, "There is none other disease to be seen in the Necke outwardly, then a swelling or tumor, which is called *Bronchocele*" (*General Practice*, p. 187).

95. Perhaps the rationale for this remedy was that the sponge would take up the fluid from the edematous tissues. Sponge was an ancient remedy for goiter; only relatively recently was it discovered that the iodine content of sponge made it of real value in this disease.

96. Some of these ingredients were considered to be astringent and hence helpful in reducing excess tissue fluid.

Observations

More thereof. Thus Mr. *Fuller* did heale divers of this dissease with applying a long time tog[ether] butter milk Curd to breake, & Flos ungent. in a plaster to heal it & diet drinks made of white wine & germander taken a long time. For purging body and bloody humours & other things [this treatment] may doe as well. [Page 155]

Legs Swollen to Cure

Lay a pickled herring to each foot 4 or 5 dayes. Or Rx. juice of wall-wort, wax, and Vinegar, barly meale. Boyl them and make a plaister. Or use oyl of swallows. In many cases such things as drive the humour into the body again is the way to destroy the boddy. In some cases only medic[ine] to strengthen the inward parts must be used. In other cases the humour must by Vessicatory or Issues or cupping be drawn out. Mind the inward cause of it principally.

Lask or Flux

Rx. of London Treacle or Mithridate the quantity of a Nutmeg, and mix it with conserve of red roses. Take the quantity of a Nutmegge before sleep. If it be extream & long continued, use bramble buds beaten and sodd in broth. Or use the infusion of Rock-Allom in white wine. If any of these help not, presently use things to purge away the cause, as Rubarb, alloes, Roses &c. [Page 156]

Loosenes

Make a Cake of wheat meale, chalk, Allom and eat it.

Steep or boyl Cranbill root or belly ake root. It cures belly ake, loosenes & griping in children & drives out bad humours; applied to soars, dries up humours. Bayberry roots boyled in water & drunk helps flux tho never so bad. Probat. est and [is an] Indian medicine.

Stamp spiders webb and Rue together. Lay on as much as a walnut on the navil. Gerry: Dr., probat. est.[97] It cures the bloody flux or any other. [Page 157]

Lice to drive away

Rx. of oyl dreggs & hoggs fatt unsalted, adde Mercury & the powder of Staves acre and annoint a woolen therewith & wear it about the middle. Or make a soft fire & put quick-silver therein & hang the lousy garments over the smoake. *Comb it near the fire for nits* [illegible].

Or take Frankincense sodd with hoggs fat, annoint where they come. Or staves acre & tobacco ashes & soap mixed together will do the like.

Observation. Occulus Indi, beaten to powder and mixed with fatt or butter doth destroy them presently. Annoynt the head &c.

Liver stopped[98]

Take chicken broth and add to it the herb Mercury & Cichory, reisins stoned & boyl them together. Blanch Almons & with the same liquor make almon milk. Let the patient drink it every morning fasting. Also the liver of a hare dried & made into fine powder is counted good for all the diseases of the liver. Also Cream of Tartar as much as will ly upon a 3d.,[99] dissolved in broth, 10 dayes together taken &c. [Page 158]

---

97. Palmer meant that a Dr. Gerry had tested this recipe.

98. Wirtzung (1617: p. 385) explains that "obstruction" of the liver occurs in its arteries and veins, thus hindering "the blood, and other humours, that should have their passage and course through the veines." Such obstruction, which may be caused by clothes that are too tight, falls, certain foods including "all manner of Pap, and other oppilating (obstructing) Pottages," cold, and so on, interferes with the proper movement of the humors and thus causes sickness.

99. A threepenny piece, a coin.

Heat of Liver

Rx. Leaves of Violets, Cinquefoil, Endive, Succory, Scabious, fumitory. These and other herbs infused in clarified whey often taken. Distilled water of strawberrys &c. [Page 159]

Lungs Inflammed or Consumption

For these in the beginning open a veine. Use Clysters and this pectoral infusion made of Liquorice, anniseed, figgs, reisins, maiden hair, Isop, sage; in 4 ounces of it add manna, 1 oz.; syr. of roses solutive, 6 drams. Use hony water, figgs, Isop, oximel.

In a hot cause,[100] Violets, the 4 great cooling seeds, french barly, maiden hair, liquorice, Isop, scabius, reysins of the sun, melon seeds.

For outward medicines Rx. fresh butter, goose grease, oyl of rue, oyl of sweet and bitter Almons, powder of orrice, Isop & horehound. Make a cerecloth &c. [Page 160]

Lungs with a Veine broken or spitting blood

Use Oximel, syr. purslaine. Bole Armeniac is very good. So is Knot-grass, Comfrey, tender leaves of Oake, pomgranate pills, blood stone, Coral, Crocus martis, Terra sigillata, drag[on's] blood, Gum arabic, frankincense, mastic, white starch, syr. of myrtles, Conserve of red roses. *But some [are] but weak. Many medicines may be made.* [Page 161]

Lungs ulcerated

It is known by spitting blood, continuall fever, salt rhume, leanne, strong Cough, difficult breathing, raising filthy matter &c.

100. That is, in lung disease due to a hot humor.

Take Rhubarb with raisens of the sun stoned every morning. Also syr. of roses solutive, broth of an ould cock with reysins and manna or cassia dissolved in it.[101]

Rx. Infusion of Colts foot, scabious, melon seeds, and 3 Cordial flours, that is Rosemary, Borage and bugloss, of each 4 oz., in which dissolve manna, 1½ oz.; syr. of violets 1 oz. Mix these and take it often. Use gentle & cooling Clysters. Then use cleansing things as hony & sugar'd water, as juice of red Coleworts, Colts foot, maiden hair, scabious, agrimony. Make [an] infusion. Adde clarifyed hony, ½ lb. Or Rx. fresh butter, 2 oz.; Turpentine, 1 oz.; English hony, 4 oz. Mix together & take what you can.

The Ulcer to heale

Rx. Conserve of roses, 4 oz.; powder of comfry roots, 1½ oz.; bole Armoniack, fox lungs alike, 2 scruples. Add syr. of myrtles. Make an electuary. Or use water of ground ivy *taken* with sugar 9 days fasting. The distilled *water* of the lungs & liver of a Calf are good. Infusion of Guajacum or China roots.

Also Lac Sulphuris & the magestery of perls & Corrall are excellent in this case. Also goats milk, asses milk, brest milk are great restoratives & continual drinking good strong beer &c. [Pages 162 and 163 are missing. Page 164]

Madnes. How cured

This is distinguished from a frenzy because a frenzy is joyned with a fever. The Cure is at first by frequent bleeding in the left arm, foot, forehead, nose. Leeches applyed behind the ears, or hemoroidial veins opened is good. Whey with syr. of Violets. Purge with Rhubarb, Senna. Epithim, polypod[ium], lapis lazuli, diagridium. This must be done several times.

Also use of Vomits. Cause sleep by use of sempervivum & poppy.

---

101. Again the treatment of like things by like things. Rhubarb (*Rheum*) should be a specific for rheumy discharges, and what creature better demonstrates healthy lungs than a long-lived rooster?

Water applyed to the forehead and head. Mandrakes are good. The head is to be washed towards night with vinagar or water. Also (its a great secret) the brains of a dogg be given boyled 3 mornings together. Also dry the roots of Nymphea gathered in May, the moon decreasing. Boyl them in wine Vinagar and bring them to powder. Give 1 dram morning and evening. Give the same in some of the Vinagar aforesaid. Also the infusion of anagallis is very good. Salt p[eter] taken often in common beer, or 10 drops of spir. of Vitrioll dropped into a pint &c. [Page 165]

Menstrual Flux

Rubb a great many shumach berrys & gett [some] of the red powder. Give 1 dram at a time. Probatum.

The bark of a White oak *or the pine nut or the staff seed. The rue or the* [illegible] *in powder stops the whites in women.*

Menstrual Flux white to stop or also the running of the reyns. Mrs. French's[?].[102] Rx. Terebinth Venetiae, 4 oz.; heartshorn, ¼ oz.; Ivory, ¼ oz.; Nutmeg, 2 drams; Cinnamon, 2 drams. Boyl thes in a sheet of white paper over a chaffin dish of coals. Give 4 pills M. & Even. *It cures the whites, running* [of] *the reins, helps terms.* Probat. est. Mrs. Baur—strew in powder.

Megrim or Vertigo

They cannot walk without staggering. He thinks the house turns round.

The cure. Let blood. Rx. Hiera picra, 2 oz., mixt with a little conserve of roses made into pills. Take 4 or 5, 3 nights together. Wash the feet with infusion of Rosemary, Cammomile, Betony &c. [Page 166]

---

102. This woman and Mrs. Baur, mentioned a few lines below, were probably midwives who gave the secret of these remedies to Palmer.

Mother

Sometimes it happeneth in women that the Matrix falleth down,[103] *and the neck, but the bladder is swollen so that* [it] *can hardly make water.* Rx. white ash bark burnt to ashes about *one* spoonfull stieped in *a half pint beer for a time: add now and then a little solid bark to all, and sometimes the bark of white ash boiled in clearing water and drink. It will cause to make water abundantly and so heal them.* Probat. est.

Rx. Burdock roots stamped & boyled in hoggs fatt. F. Empl. with bees wax &c. S.A. Apply *to* the navil, *cutting a hole for the navel to come through.*[104]

Emplastrum Hystericum to settle the Mother & keep it in its place[105] & stop the fitts of it from either rising to high or falling too low. Spread on leather or thick linnen cloth in this form. Place the navil through the hole to make a plaister.[106]

Rx. Maudlin, Mugwort, Burdock leaves & roots, Carrot Seed, double tansy, mother time, Featherfew, Galbanum, taccamahac, Assafoitida, Bedellium, Castoreum, Myrrh, Musk, Nutmegs, Cinnamon, cloves, Bees-wax, Bayberry-wax, Turpentine, ship-pitch, Rozin melted & the other ingredients powdered & sifted. F. Emp. S.A. [Page 167]

Mouth Ulcers

In Infants they are cured with mouth waters of plantain, sage, Cinquefoil, burnt Allom, hony. Or Rx. infusion of Galls that Ink is made with; being strained, add honey. In old or grevious [cases], open a Veine, apply Cupping glasses to the Neck with scarrifica-

103. Falling of the mother, or matrix, was prolapse of the uterus.

104. This instruction is followed by a sketch of a crescent-shaped bandage with a hole in the center. Evidently the ointment was to be spread on the bandage and the latter was to be applied to the abdomen.

105. It was believed that the uterus, when disturbed, wandered about in the abdomen, causing various symptoms including hysteria. *Rising of the mother* produced a feeling of suffocation.

106. See n. 104.

tion.[107] Bleed under the Tongue. Wash the mouth with infusion of sumach, Vine leaves, plantain, purslain, pomegranate pills, Vinagr., Diamoron or Dianucum, powder of orange pills, mixed hony and Allom. Or take the spir. of Vitriol mixed with hony & burnt Allom. If the ulcers be very foul, Rx. Verdegreese, 1 dram; Allom, ½ oz.; white Copperas, 1 dram. Boyl these in white wine, 4 oz. Add Aqu. vit. Wash the mouth therewith.

Soar Mouth. Mouth Ulcer

Use gentle purges. Also syr. vitr, 2 drops [in] a spoonful of hony. Filthy soars in the mouth must be cured with strong medicines. Rx. Verdegreese, 1 dram; Allom ½ oz.; vitriol, [illegible], of each 1 dram in white wine infusion, 4 oz.; Aqua vita, 1 oz. With this touch the soar, but take heed of swallowing any down, & spitt it out. Burnt fennel roots & hony. Annoynt if ulcer spreads.

Pallet of the Mouth down

Rx. Rosemary, cummin-seed, bay salt. Tye them up in a ragg together and lay to the nape of the neck; bind it too with a fillet. [Page 168 is blank. Page 169]

Melancholy in extremity. How Cured.

Rx. Senna, 2 oz.; Anniseed prepared in small beer or whey. Take of it many days together. Or for a preparative take Tartar Vitriolate ten days together. For a purge, Rx. extract of black hellebore, 1 scruple or ½ dram. It will be good to open veines of the nose, Temples, Forehead or behind the Ears. Also sneezing powder is good in this case.

107. Scarification: the making of numerous small, superficial incisions, done to promote bleeding.

Ŗ: White ash bark burnt to
ashes, about — spoonfull steep'd

Ŗ: Burdock roots [...] boos ma[...]
So: As apply [...] y.e navil [...]

Emplastrum Hystericum, to settle y.e
mother, & keep it in it's place, & hinders fits of it
from either rising so [...] or falling too, low:
spread on leather, or thick lining cloth, on th[...]
form, place the navil thro the hole,
to make y.e plaister —
Ŗ: Motudlin, Mugwort, Burdock, leavs & roots,
carrot seed, double tansy, mother thime, Feathe[...]
Galbanum, Assafætida, Bdellium, Myrrh, Mast[...]
Nutmegs, Cinnamon, cloves, Bees-wax, Bay-be[...]
— wax, Turpentine, Ship-pitch, Rosin, & y.e other
ingredients, powderd & sifted F: Empl: S.A. ——

Mouth Ulcers.

In Infants they are cured with mouth waters.
of Plantain Sage Cinqufoil, burnt Allom,
&y. or ℞. ℥ of Galls ʒ. Ink is made with
being strained and honey. In elder persons
upon a Veine, apply Cupping glasses to ye Neck
with Scarrification. Blood under the Tongue &
wash ye mouth wt. ℥ of Sumach, Vine Leaves
plantain purslain, pomgranate pills & Vineg:
Diamoron or Dianucum. powder of orange
pills. mixed hony and allom. or take ℥ of
℥ Vitriol mixed wt. hony & burnt allom. If
the ulcers be very foul ℥ Verdegreace ℥
allom ℥ſſ. white ℥ſſ Vitriol ʒj Royl steep in white
wine ℥iiij add dyt vit. wash the mouth therewith

Soar Mouth. Mouth Ulcers.

ye gentle purges. also ʒ℞. Vitr. gutt. 2
a spoonfull of hony. filthy soars in the
mouth must be cured wt. strong medicines
℞. Verdegreace ʒj allom ℥ſſ. Vitriol & white
wine ʒj bin white wine ℥℥iiij. Roꝛe pyll
℥j. with this touch the soar. But take heed
of swallowing any down, & spit it out. burnt
sinart roots & hony. Annoynt if ulcers

Pallet of the Mouth down.
℞. Rosemary Cumin-seed bay salt. wrt these
up in a ragg together and lay to the nape of
the neck. bind it too with a fillot. — — —

Hypocondrical Melancholly, how cured

The Melancholly is seated in the Hypocondrium in the liver and spleen, especially in the stomach & Midriff or missenteary. *In milt this melancholy is seated.* Signes: [1.] sadnes without cause, sudden fears & strong Imaginations without grounds, the last only for a time. 2. a singing in the ears, a noise & mumbling in the head. Darknes in the sight & all things turning round. 3. Trembling heart. 4. Want of sleep. 5. Sometimes fainting fitts and swooning. 6. A bad stomach not able to digest & the body much bound (constipated).

Use lenitive clysters & phlebotomy in the Hemoroidal veines with Leeches. Open a veine in the arm in strong bodys. Use Vomits and wormwood wine or bark 30 or 40 dayes together with Tamarisk, Sassaparilla infused therein. Above all steels pills give excellent [illegible]. [Page 170]

Rx. Steele prepared, 2 drams; species diarodon abbatis, aloes, of each 1 oz.; with syrup of maiden hair. F. Pill. Let the pty (party) take 4 or 5 small pills 20 or 30 days together & unless steele goes down by stool[108] (which may appear by the blacknes of the stoole) let the party take pills of Aloes, of roses, or pills de tribus every 4 (fourth) day. After these pills taken every day an hour, take a draught of whey made of Goats milk. Take dayly oximel of Squills a spoonfull or two after you have been in use of these pills. [Page 171]

Nipples soar

Rx. oyl of hazel-nuts pressed out between a pair of hott tongues (tongs) *in* Celandine Wild, Stew'd in Cream. [Pages 172–73 are missing. Page 174 is blank. Page 175]

Palsy, Dead Palsy & Cure

Sometimes a part is dead, sometimes a whole side & sometimes all the lower parts from the hips. Caused of phlegm[109] *some times.*

108. Unless the steel from the pills is eliminated in the stools.
109. Caused by an excess of phlegm, one of the four humors. The medications that Palmer now suggests were intended to clear the body of it.

Use gentle purges and Clysters. Rx. pill. Asaserath, 1½ drams; alophangia, agric. (agaric) troch[es], of each 1 dram; mastic, 1 scruple;
cum Syr. Stoechas, simpl. vel ex scillit. F. Pill. Take 1 dram at a
time. Or use pill. Hira (hiera) picra. Use Vomits often. Use medicines
dayly that hath Caster distel. You may use pill. de agaric, Cochia
Fetida, de Hermodact, de sagapene, Hira logadii, Hira pachii, es-
pecial[ly] pill. de Iva & these often repeated.
Also use conserve of primrose mixed with mithridate. Sneezing
powders & masticatorys taken fasting are good. Sweating is good
with sassafras, guaiacum, sassaparilla, sage nutmegs & rosemary, his
ordinary drink [being] made of China roots in fair water. Cupping
glasses to the part affected. Use outwardly oyle of worms, oyle of
peper, oyl of foxes, oyl of Vipers. [Page 176 is blank. Page 177]

Plague or Pestilence

Rx. of Rue & Sage, of each.[110] Boyl it in 3 pints of Malmsey or
Muscadine or Sack till a pint be wasted. Set it over the fire again.
Adde to it long pepper Ginger, small beaten. Let them boyle a little,
put in Mithridate, 4 scruples; of London Treacle, 2 scruples. Add
to it good aqua Vitae & strong Angelica water. It must be taken
warm, a spoonfull or 2 M. & E. & so sweat thereon & if it come
freely due not force it. This alone will help by Gods blessing.
Also infusion of Garlic in milk. Also *waters of* Angelica, Mithridate
Dragon water, water of Carduus Benedictus.
Beware of catching cold in or after sweating in pestilential Diseases, for it is exceeding perilous. [Page 178 is blank. Page 179]

Pleurisies

Sometimes in the right side, sometimes in the left, it is attended
with a Cough & difficult breathing or a fever.
Rx. The pouder of the Dried pizle of a Dear or the pouder of the
jawbone of a Pike. Drink it in Carduus posset drink. Or apply out-

110. The amount has been crossed out.

wardly, to the place over medicined rags.[111] Open a Veine in the
arm on the contrary side as often as occasion requires.

N.B. Pouder of Goats blood prepared, 1 dram, given in wine a
present remedy. A julep of stone horse dung steeped in wine & the
wine *taken* 2 or 3 times & sweating much is profitable. [Page 180]

Pissing blood

Camonomile (camomile), Agrimony, Shepheards purse, Knot-grass,
Horsetail boyled in white wine.

Opopanax des[pumata], 1 dram, corrected with mastick & dissolved in Vinagar. [Page 181]

Pox. Small Pox & Meazells

The Measels are only red spots in the skin & are less dangerous.

The small pox begins with great paine in the back & head & great
sleepines in any time & is a common disease. The cure of this is to
open a veine before the 4th day & before spotts appear. If the body
be bound at the beginning, a gentle purge of syrup of roses & senna
or Cassia is good, but commonly all purging medicines are to be
avoided, especially in children, & when the body is not extreemly
bound. If nature work kindly it is better to leave the whole cure to
nature.

If the Pox[112] come slowly out,[113] some Cordialls must be given to
expell them. Use roots & seeds of fennell, Card. Ben., burn[t]
maiden-hair, broth of red peas, scordium, scabious, myrhh, especially figgs, Treacle, Mithridate, Saffron, heartshorn. All cooling
medicines are to be avoided, especially after they break out.

Or Take of Figgs *also*, raisens stoned, 2 oz.; fennel seed, 3 drams;
saffron, 1 scruple; Gum Tragacanth, 3 drams. Let the infusion be
in 3 pints of water till a 3rd part be consumed. Drink 3 or 4 ounces

---

111. Palmer does not say what medicine was to be put on the rags.

112. Palmer uses *pox* to refer both to the disease and to the *pocks*, the characteristic
lesions.

113. If the pocks appear slowly.

at a time fasting. Give to Children figgs to eat. Gum Lacca is as good as Tragacanth in this Dissease.

It is good to defend divers parts of the body. To defend Lungs take syr[up] of poppy & Colts foot, or Jujubes or Violets, Conserve of Roses, Tragacanth.

To defend the Gutts use syrup of Quinces, myrtles, rice twice boyled in plantain water and plantain seeds.

To defend the eyes & face use our medicined raggs. Also rose *water* or plantain *water*, a little saffron are good.

To defend the nostrills *with*, wash them with Vinagar or roses. If the eyes be shutt up with the nose, wash them with warm milk or infusion of Linseed or fenul (fennel) root. Drop into the ears oyl of roses or Myrtles.

To keep the throat use [Page 182] Gargarisms of the infusion of prunella, plantain, roses, balust with the juice of sharp pomgranats, syr[up] of Mirtles, hony or roses, Diacorum, Diacodium[?]. Outwardly apply to the throat our medicined rags.

If the ears be pained, dip a spunge with warm water mixed with oyl of violets. Lay this to the ears.

Sometimes the Nostrills are stopped with the pox. To help, let the party stuff up oxicratum or the Vapour of the infusion of red roses, plantain, bramble bud, willow leaves, Vine branches, or the infusion of some of these.

The Pox that continues raw, long & hard, it will be good to ripen them with the Vapour of water wherein Camomile hath been decocted. Or foment & bath them with infusion of the flours of mallow roses & figgs. Take heed of scratching the pox if you would avoid scarrs. If the pox be many and great, especially knotted together, it is good to open them after the 7th day of the appearing, which is the 11th day of the dissease, but they must not be clipped but opened with a needle.

To dry up the pox sprinkle upon them the powder of Frankincense, mastic and myrhh. The marks of the pox may be holpen thus. Wash the places with infusion of lupin peas or beans or barly, tansy, centaury, the lesser Celandine, juice of Lemmons, soap with Nitre.

To fill up the pitts, man's fatt is commended & the fatt of the fish Ascia. The sick person must be carefully kept from the cold air &

from much heat. If the first 4 days, let the patient abstain from eggs
& fresh broth. Use thin diet of easy digestion. The stomach should
be forced to eat something. Also raw fruits must be avoided & especially summer fruits because they soon turn to putrifaction. Avoid
wine and drink small beer warm instead thereof & it will be good.
So Quench a Gad of Iron or [Page 183] steele in it. Too much sleep
or watching is bad. If the party be much costive, use sometimes,
though seldom, gentle enema & glandule.[114] [Page 184]

Physick. Rx. Salat Oyl, a Gill; Sperma Ceti, a Gill; Hony, a Gill;
Rum, a Gill; Spirit of Sulphur per campanum, quarter of an ounce.
Mix. Take night and morning upon the point of a knife.[115] [Page
185]

The Purples

The cure hereof may be purchased[116] with the infusion against
the Plague. They (purples) are known by the red spots upon the
skin like flea-biting. Only flea-bitings have a prick in the middle,
which these spotted fevers & purples have not.

For the Cure, first use a gentle purge of manna, Syrup of roses
solutive, Cream of Tartar, or Pill. Pestilentiales, 1 dram. Or Rx.
sorrel, ½ minim; Card[uus] Ben[edictus], Scordium, of each 1 part;
senna, ½ dram; Rubarb, ½ dram; Citron seed, Cinnamon, of each
1 scruple; Cordial flours, 1 part. Infuse them in a quart of water,
then dissolve manna, ½ oz.; syr[up] of roses solutive, ½ oz.; spir[itus]
Vitr., 2 drps. Vomits are good.

In strong bodys open a Vein before the 4th day. Sweats are good
in this case. Or take the seeds of Marrow or napus, 1 dram; of [il-
legible], Card. ben., of each ½ dram; Card. water, 4 oz. Make an
emulsion. Add syr. of Scordium, ½ oz., powder of harts horn, scabious water & London treacle; bezor, 3 grains.

---

114. A glandule enema was intended to benefit the glandules, the little swellings
of smallpox.
115. Take as much as can be carried on the point of a knife.
116. Achieved.

If a looseness happen in this case it is dangerous, but it may not be stopped except it be extream. That must be done with Treacle or conserve of roses. Use Alkermes in sorrel or Strawberry water. Also unguents or oyles of Scorpions are good. Also Vesicatorys are profitable in those that are outwardly cold or inwardly hot, that is, very hot, & when the head is afflicted & and sence and reason troubled. Also a posset made with purple grass is pretious. [Page 186]

Poisons Taken

How Cured

Signs of Poison taken: 1. Change of the Colour of the face to black or yellow. 2. frequent vomiting. 3. swooning fitts frequently with cold sweats.

Signs of hot poison

[1.] Excess of heat in the mouth, Throat, stomach, Gutts, great thirst & sweat. 2. Sometimes Corrosion & paines intollerable in the inward parts. 3. Vomiting. 4. Sweats. 5. Swooning & sudden deaths.

Signs of Cold Poison

1. Heavy, sleepy & drowsy. 2. Convultions in the Eyes, mouth, arms & leggs. 3. Face ghastly. 4. The body benummed.

As soon as it is percieved the poison is taken, its good presently to vomit with water & oyl mixed together, taken warm, or butter dissolved in warm oyl a good quantity. If the party cannot vomit, purge the Aloes & Rubarb. Also use fatt clysters with butter & Cows milk & the muscilage of linseed.

N.B. It is a generall Rule, that the poison should be driven away the same way it is taken. As taken by the mouth, by Vomiting. By the nose, by sneezing. At the fundament, by Clysters. If outward, by revulsions. Strong ligatures about the arms & leggs. So are cupping glasses [also effective].

Cure of particular poisons. Mandrake that causeth sleep is cured by eating radish seeds with bread and salt. Also by sneezing [Page

187] and by the infusion of coriander or peneroyal in fair water oft given. Opium [poisoning] is cured by Castorium, 2 drams, given in urine. Hemlock is cured by Vomits and Clysters. Also Treacle is good. Cantharides taken inwardly are cured with Vomits & Clysters made with infusion of mallows, french barly, fenucreek seed, Linseed, oyle of Lillys, goat's suet. Also Treacle, milk, juice of lettuce is good.

In like manner are cured the poisons of Arsnick, Sublimate, Ver. Oris & litharge is cured by a Vomit & afterwards by pigeons dung, beer or urine &c. to drink. Arsnick is cured by the oyl of pine Kernells speedily given. Take 1 lb., then procure Vomiting. Then give milk to drink & Clysters of the same. Unquencht lime & auripigmentum is cured with fatt things & lenitive potions by the infusions of Linseed, marshmallows, aqua & hony & wine. [Page 188]

Quinsey

Rx. Hony of roses, ½ oz.; oyl of Turpentine, 2 drams; oyl of cinnamon, 6 drops; dust of crabb's claws, 3 grains; oyl of Vitriol, 4 drops. Of all which mixt & beat together give inwardly eight or 12 drops & Annoint outwardly under the end of the jaw bones. Let blood also under the tongue if the person be capable.[117] *This cures any quinsy or trouble in the third day. A French doctor's recept but cured many.* [Page 189]

Rupture or Burstnes

Rx. Plantain, roses, Comfry, greater & lesser young fern especially of the first springing up, avens, Valerian, horstail, Vervain, of each 1 minim; Liver wort, 2 minims; Nutmegs, Cinnamon, Corrall, white bread, of each ½ oz.; hony, half a pint. Add sumach, bruscus roots. It will be more available (effective) if you make it with Comfry & the tops of young fern brewed in your beer.

Besides use this plaister. Rx of Comfry roots, 1 oz.; red roses, bean meale, of each ½ oz. Let all be brought to dust & mixed with

117. If the patient is strong enough.

Goats fatt. Ad some wax & make an unguent. Renew this every day for many days together. There may be added bears fat. *But before the application put this* [*on*], *or before* a new medicine is to be laid on, use fomentations of Comfry roots, Solomons Seale, red roses, shepperds pouch, plantain, mouse ear, horstail, roots of tormentil, allom or the bark of Frankencense boyled soft & immediately annoint the back with oyl of Hypericon or oyl of turpentine.

Also thorowax alias perfoliata is of singular use, either outwardly or inwardly taken, but if these or the like medicines avail not, then the patient must continually wear a truss.

There be windy, watry & fleshy ruptures. Besides the rupture at the Codd, there is the rupture at the navel or below. Vid. Hernia.[118] [Page 190 is blank. Page 191]

Sciatica and Cure

It is a grevious pain in the hips or the bone called Sciatica (ischiadic) bone.

Give 1 dram of Pulvis Arthriticus for a purge taken fasting. Betimes in the morning after, bleed in the foot on the side pained. Apply a Cupping glass to the hip or in want of it, a dish with smooth brims. Boyl it well in water & cover the brim of the dish with a double cloth & so slap it speedily upon the hip dry and hold it on a quarter of an hour. This will make a blyster and fetch of [off] the skin.[119] After[ward] annoint the part with basilicon & draw it with Cabbage leaves as long as it will run & so heale it. Use baths & sweats with Guajacum, Sassaparilla. Use plasters of pitch & brimstone. [Page 192]

118. Wirtzung (pp. 276–77) says that of the ruptures into the cod or scrotum, the "three chief ones are caused of swelling, of scabbines, or of striving" (straining). He adds that these may be produced by wind (intestinal gas), by varices, by descent of the intestine or omentum "into the cod"—that is, by an inguinal hernia—and by water. If a rupture, adds Wirtzung, "proceed of wind, that may be heard by the shreeking or rumbling"—that is, by borborygmus, the sounds made by intestinal gas. These are indeed diagnostic, but the rupture is not caused by gas.

119. As the heated cupping glass or dish, its mouth tightly applied to the skin, cools, a partial vacuum develops inside the vessel, and the enclosed epidermis separates—is "fetched off"—producing a kind of blister.

Soars that be ould

A strong infusion of white oak bark with sage and Allom. For new soars use it without the sage & Allom. *Aliud.* Rx. Copperas burnt upon an Iron shovle. Then boyle it in water and use only that water to wash it. Rx. Willow root bark by poultis or decoction dries humours in weeping, running soars. Or the bark laid to the soar. Probat. est. [Page 193]

Spleen & the obstruction thereof[120]

Signs: great heavines in left side, below the short ribbs, afterwards paine especially in running or walking a pace. Also difficult breathing, a drie Cough, palpitation of the heart & a greedy appitite.

Take as much Cream of Tartar in broth every morning as will ly upon a 3 pence, especially Cream of Tartar Vitriolate. Use steele pills, oximell of squills & drink made with Tamariske. Also Vomiting is good. So is the infusion or water of bugloss, and so is Treacle.

Or Rx. Germander, Isop, rosemary, Centaury, of each 1 minim; Tamariske barke, sassafras, of each 2 drams. Boyle all this in your beer & drink of it dayly at Fall & Spring.

Or *make so.* Sow up all the particulars (ingredients) in a bag, infuse them in wine & drink every morning a draught. Ol. anisii & ol. succini, equal drops. Very profitable.

Outwardly to the region of the Spleen, take henbane leaves sod in Vinagar & ol. Capparib. & lay them on hott for a fomentation. Then take broom flours, 2 minims. Let them be sodd & bruised in a close Vessel. Ad thereto Dialthea, 2 oz.; Armoniack dissolved in Vinagar. Lay on this plaster. Or dissolve armoniack in Vinagar, spread it on lether & apply it. Also oyl of Capers or Rue or bitter Almons, especially the armoniack plaister aforesaid. [Page 194]

---

120. Culpeper explains that the "Spleen takes the thickest or Melancholly blood to it self" (*Pharmacopoeia*, pp. 280–81). From such blood comes both black bile and melancholy humor; he distinguishes between the two. In obstruction of the spleen, the two must be purged from the organ.

Spleen swelling

A sensible (perceptible) swelling in the left side & from thence paine. The spleen, being pressed, somewhat yields & together a rumbling is heard & sometimes unsavoury belchings. This comes many times from wind & windy meats. Use manna, Cassia, Syr. roses, afterwards infusion of Cammomile flours in sack. Or Diaciminum or Diacalaminth. Troches of Capers are good. Outwardly use fomentations of the bark of Capers, Tamarisk flours, leaves of rue, Calamint, Mellilote, Cummin seed. Bay berries are good, sodd in water & Vinagar. After(ward) annoynt the part with oyl of rue or bays or capers. A Cupping glass to spleen good.[121]

Inflamation of the Spleen

A great heat on the left side, with a swelling & the left Kedny is pained together with it, and there goes a palpitation, beating or trembling with it, a Continual fever, & difficult breathing.

First open a Veine in the left arm or the Hemorrhoids veines may be opened.[122] Annoint the spleen with Vinagar & oyl of roses mixed together. Also a gentle purge with the lenitive electuary or Diacatholicon & syr. roses solutive & Cream of tartar. Then take meale of [Page 195] beans & barly, powder of wormwood and cammomile, 2 oz.; oyl of roses, saffron a little. Make it into a plaister. Apply it.

Schyrhus of the Spleen

Rx. Armoniack dissolved in Vinagar & strained, 1 dram.; aloes ros., 2 drams; pil. de tribus, ½ dram; salt of wormwood & ash, 2 scruples; oyl of Anniseed, 4 grains. Make pills & give 1 scruple or scruples. Then take the roots or wood of Tamarisk, boyl it in clean smith's water & drink of this.

Outwardly apply Mallows, Mars-mallows, figgs, lilly roots, Chamomile flours, rue leaves, mustard seeds. Also Armoniack dissolved in Vinagar, Diachilon simple & compound, Dialthea, especially

121. Without scarification, a heated cupping glass was applied to the skin over the spleen as a form of counterirritation.
122. See n. 60.

Hemlock and Armoniack dissolved in Vinagar. Also take a Spunge filled with the water of quick limes and apply it to the Spleen.[123] [Page 196 is blank. Page 197]

Scalding. vid. Burning[124]

Stomach paines & wind in Bowels. Take long pepper, Cumin seeds, Calamus, Bay berrys, and let them be in fine powder of each a like quantity. Boyl them in hony to a confection. The dose is the quantity of a nutmeg.

Aliud. Rx. Angelica & Alicampane & gentian roots & seeds of fennel or Caraway. Make a decoction in water in a pint of the liquour. Dissolve 2 drams of salt of angelica. Take S (several?) spoonfulls at a time, 3 times a day.

Sinews & their shrinking[125]

Oyl of Hypericon, oyl of Foxes, Nerve oyl, oyl of earthworms, [oil of] serpents, scorpions. Or take the marrow of a hors-bone and elder Crops, sage, 2 minims, boyld in the marrow. Add hony a spoon full, aqua vitae a spoonful, a little pepper & boyl it again. Keep it for use.

Or take neets foot oyl, 2 parts; bullocks gaul (gall), one part; aqua vitae and rose water, 2 spoonfulls. [Page 198]

Scabs. see Itch

Scald Heads

Rx. Water, 2 lbs.; Alom, ½ oz.; hony, a pint; scum (skim) it clean in boyling. Add to it Vir. Oris, 2 drams. Boyl it & filtre it & use it.

123. The external application of medications in cases of "schyrhus," or cancer, of the spleen again illustrates the belief that medicines could be absorbed through the skin and find their way to an internal organ.

124. This heading means that for the treatment of scalding the reader should see the section on burns. Palmer now discusses the "scalding" of gastric pain.

125. *Sinew* could mean tendon or nerve. The symptoms of this "shrinking" are not described. Palmer may have had in mind what is now called tenosynovitis, painful inflammation of the tendon and its sheath, or cramp, or some form of neuralgia.

Or take lye, 2 lbs.; white wine, 1 lb.; merc[ury] sublimate, 1 dram; s[alt] peter, 2 oz. Boyl them & being wasted, filtre it & use it.

Swelling, hot, to scatter & disperse

Rx. Celandine, plantain, sorrel & boyl them in Cream till it comes to an oyl and strain them out.[126] [Page 199]

Stone

A certain Gentleman in England was cured of the stone by taking for several weeks this medicine. Rx. White wine, a pint; mise (mice) dung beaten, two spoon fulls. Boyl it in the wine till it be wasted half. Take a spoonful or two at a nines (nine o'clock?), following it several days & weeks if need requires.

Item Rx. Cammomile, Agrimony, Shepheards grass, Knot-grass, Hors-tail, boyled in white wine. Good for the stone, strangury, pissing of blood &c.

Item. Opopanax, 1 dram, corrected with mastick & dissolved in Vinagar. [Page 200]

Terms to stop

Shepherds-purse, strawberries, Water-lillies, plantaine, House-leek, Comfrey, Knot-grass, Solomon-Seale roots. Also these are good against pissing blood.

Rx. Soft hoggs dung applyed before & behind, i.e., to the small of her back & to her belly below. It will put a stop to the immoderate & excessive overflowing of the terms in women with child; it may be safely used &c. Probat. est. [Page 201]

Terms to provoke

Garlick, Maidenhair, Mugwort, Wormwood, Betony, Centaury, Cammomile, Calaminth, Dodder, Fennel, St. Johnswort, Marjoram,

---

126. Culpeper says that plantain and sorrel are cooling and drying, while celandine is heating (*Pharmacopoeia*, pp. 4, 10, 16). Thus this prescription seems confused in terms of humoral theory.

Horehound, Bawm, Water-cresses, Origanum, Peniroyal, parsly, smallage, Rue, Rosemary, Sage, Savin, Time, Mother-time, Nettles. [Page 202 is blank. Page 203]

Vomiting & Loosnes in Children

Andromachus Treacle[127] mixed with mel rosarum. Proved. Or give a vomit while they (the sick children) have strength of nature to bear it. I gave a Vomit of Crocus *to one of my ch*[*ildren*] [*this same color*][128] of a year & a quarter old. In this case, it helped by God's blessing presently. A sutable dose of sulphur of Antimony[129] rightly prepared [is] a good help in this case before the child be farr spent. [Page 204]

Urine to move

Rx. Couch grass seed stamped and boyled in spring water with maiden-hair and marigold flowers. Probatus est.

Rx. Dried grasshopper, ½ dram. A great secret. So is powder of Niter & sal prunella, [a] present remedy.

Rx. White ash bark ashes steeped in beer & drunk. Item. Calam. Aromat.[130] in pouder *or the* Salt *of it,* ½ dram; *put the powder that rubbeth off in them to provoke, turn* (relieve) *and heal the lungs and* remove new phlegm and ill humours.

Rue dryed in pouder & taken in white dinner cyder, Agrimony, hartychoaks (artichokes), read (red) betony, plantain, winter Cher-

---

127. *Treacle* sometimes meant molasses, but here it refers to theriac, an almost incredible mixture made from seventy-two ingredients including opium and viper's flesh. Theriac was an ancient remedy against poison, particularly that of a venomous snake. Theriaca Andromachi, the theriac of Andromachus the Elder (fl. 60 A.D.), physician to the Emperor Nero, had been modified by Andromachus from an earlier prescription of Mithridates (120–63 B.C.). By Palmer's time the Theriaca Andromachi contained a mere sixty-five or so ingredients (Culpeper, *Pharmacopoeia*, pp. 166–67).

128. Of the same color, that is, a solution of the same concentration.

129. *Crocus metallorum*, q.v.

130. *Calamus aromaticus* was a remedy for diseases of the lungs as well as for difficult urination.

ries, horstail, hysop, fennel & parsly roots; pouder of Rubarb in plantain water.

Also Violets, Mallows & the four greater seeds. Also use Turpentine & apply astringent things. *In a* hot cause[131] use marjoram. These provoke Urine & are good for pissing of blood.

Rx. Pouder of egg shells, spruse turpentine, sorrel seed. F. pilul. *or take therein* (internally). Help the diseases of the milt *and such stomachs as* loath *their* meat.

Rx. Terebint. cocta, ½ oz., Rhubarb. electissimi, 3 drams; succini albi, succi glycyrr., of each ½ dram; Cinamo electi, 1 dram. S.a., f. pil. *Give them at will. Be still and it will provoke urine.*

Rx. Broom seed: it potently provokes Urine & breakes the stone.

Rx. Pulv. Testis Apri. It clenseth the bladder, causeth to make urine. Give dos(e) as much as will ly on a 6*d.* or shilling. [Page 205]

Whites in Women

Vid. Menstrua alba, pag. 165[132] [Page 209][133] D. (Dr.) Brattle's Directions for Joseph Bowen's Child. Salt of [illegible], 1 scruple; Powders of Ethiops mineral, 6 grains in a powder. Two Powders a day with syrup of Elderberrys. One Purge a week for three weeks.

Rx. powdered Gallap (jalap). Crem. tartar. Calomel mixed [illegible] 3 grains to be taken in [illegible]. Make a strong Decoction of sassafras Bark. Put a Gallon of the Decoction on [illegible] unslaked Lime [illegible] as to Dissolve. Let it remain 24 hours, then decant & bottle. Half a pint in 24 hours to be taken. [Page 210][134]

A Water from the Root of Angelica, *or steeped in* [*a*] *pan and distilled;* 2 or 3 spoonfulls at a time easeth all paines & Torments coming of

131. If the stoppage is due to heat.
132. Of pages 206–19, which should follow in Palmer's notebook, only six pages, one of them blank, had been photocopied. The numbers for these are almost illegible because of foxing. Presumably the pages missing from the photographic copy were all blank. Regular pagination begins again at page 220.
133. Not in Palmer's hand.
134. This and the following pages are again in Palmer's hand. On page 204 he had reached the Ws and the end of his alphabetical listing of ailments. What now follows is a miscellany of information he wanted to remember.

cold wind, the bad [illegible] not being bound, & the same water
taken with the powder or the root of Angelica at first helps pleurisy,
diseases of the lungs & brest cough. The physick [helps] short
breathing.[135] Syrup of the stalks doth the like.

This water for paine of Collick, strangury, stopping urine, procures Courses stopped,[136] helps after-birth, for liver & spleen, discusses all windines & inward swellings. *I believe (thus* Mr. *Fuller) if
the water be stoppered in* [illegible]. *But beer or cider or honey new distilled
doth as well as wine.*

You may add to the spirit salt of Wormwood or of peneroyal or
Alicampane or other chymicall salts.

Take Marine or Nitrus salt either together or apart by themselves
and put into a retort with a receiver.[137] Then with the heat of fire
distill a sour & sharp mercurial liquor. Then with a greater heat
cometh forth a salt sulphurus and nitrus and sweet. The third re-
maineth in the bottom fixed. Here is a mistery for the Learned to
improve. [Several missing, presumably blank pages. Page 217]

A Body Compounded out of [illegible] Hypostatical beginnings,
namely Sal, Sulphur and Mercury, as is hereafter taught, called a
Quintessence, an Elixar & universal Medicine.[138]

Behold then how a perfect & universal medicine is prepared out
of all things in Nature whether vegetable, animal or mineral. Neither
is there anything more easy than preparation thereof, especially out
of Herbs and plants, so that no labour ought to be omitted in the
preparations of medicines after this manner. For these medicines
are wholy free from those dropsy (watery) substances that the gen-
erality of other medicines are filled withall, that hinders both good
to the patient and Comfort to the physitian.

135. Shortness of breath.
136. Restores menstruation.
137. At this point the author turns to general and philosophical remarks on the
nature and basic elements of medicines, their modes of action, the origins of disease,
and related topics. He begins with the Paracelsian concept that man's spirit, soul,
and body are associated with the three basic principles, the *tria prima:* mercury,
sulphur, and salt, which also represent water, air, and earth.
138. Although a plant, for example, includes "hypostatical" or druglike material,
from it may be extracted the vital salt, sulphur, and mercury. From these three may
be compounded a quintessence, or elixir, the perfect and universal medicine.

Also of those medicines a few drops will be sufficient with God's ordinary blessing. Also these medicines do comfort and revive the spirits and I am sure that is the best way to encounter with any distemper. Observe also by the way that man's nourishment of his body is by the spirits (nutritive elements) of his food that is separated both in the stomach and Veines and all the dropsy part is expelled out of the body by seige, by sweat, by urine & other wayes.[139]

Then surely a true Physitian must be an Imitatour of Nature in the separation of all the excremonial (worthless) & unprofitable part of his medicine, before such time as his patient recover. But how this is to be done very few do know, & some that do know it by reason of impediments cannot attend to it. But no man shall proceed any further than divine providence permits.

But to return to the universal medicine; I shall insert what the [Page 218] Learned speake of it. It is a Universal cleanser, a universal healer, a Universal emptier of all impuritys. This medicine is made of a fixed Salt, and a Flying Volatile salt, called a mercurial Salt, that is remaining in the distilled water of a plant, that has a strong tast of the plant. I say these forementioned salts must be brought into a body with the proper natural oyl of the plant, the true spirit of wine being added thereunto.[140] The heat of the oyl is taken away with the sharpnes of the Salt, and the sharpnes of the salt is taken away with the tast of the oyl. This is that medicinal Balsam that does revive our nature and radical balsam.[141] Whereas most of the medicines of other physitians, they are yet Crude, impure and gross, and are clogged with terrestrial thicknes. They rather clogg and overlay nature before she can extract their maligne quality, concoct their crudity & drive in the early grossness & impurity, the which being a task-burden (an assigned burden), she fainteth before she can re-

139. Just as the vital principles may be extracted from a plant, leaving behind the impurities, so man's stomach and veins separate the nutritive elements from his food. The useless residue is eliminated.

140. The ideal medicine, a universal healer and cleanser, consists of fixed salt (sulphur) and volatile salt (mercury) combined with the essential oil of the plant.

141. The essence of the plant was sometimes called "radical" because it was the fundamental or "root" substance of the plant.

ceive any help or comfort.[142] But yet, friendly Reader, if thou hast the best medicines in the World, how easily can God take away the Vertue, and yet on the other side (hand) we must not expect that [virtue] in the things which God hath not furnished them with [at] all, *as for example to few on earth, though it should enrich the body or beget and recover bliss and spirits when they are wasted and decayed.*

The Reason why many fall short of the Benefits of Medicine [Page 219]

Know that Sin is the Cause of all Diseases, and sometimes Diseases are immediately sent by God, and he alone must take them away by himself without instrumental means.[143]

2 ly (Secondly), oftentimes they come by some disorder of the patient, and they are ordinarily humoural distempers. Sometimes people think the strength of nature will drive it out, [delaying] till it is too late.[144] Sometimes people are not willing to be at charge (to undergo expense for medical treatment) and follow their own apprehensions (understanding) and the apprehensions of those that have no real knowledge, skill nor judgment and think much to learn. Sometimes [it is] the wickednes & covetousness of some that profess skill [so] that many are afraid to trust them.

Sometimes the slighting and undervaluing of those [physicians] they know, and running [instead] after strangers, especially those that have a flattering tongue, brave show, and will promise that which is in no man's power to perform. Sometimes going to the physitian, but not to God, as Asa did,[145] and so incurr the danger of that curse [which] belongs to those that trust in an arm of flesh. Sometimes the wilfulnes of some that will not be ruled by those [physicians] they make choice of but will goe from one to another

142. The impurities of ordinary medicines, not prepared with care, overwhelm the body of the sick patient before any value can be extracted from them.

143. That is, only God can cure some diseases.

144. Now Palmer catalogues the reasons why some sick persons fail to seek competent treatment.

145. "And Asa did that which was right in the eyes of the Lord, as did David his father" (1 Kings 15:11).

without ground or reason, and contrary to reason & honesty except their physician desire it,[146] or have wholly left them, or apparently administer that which is unsutable or unsafe for their present condition [and] malady.

Lastly, the want of knowledge in the physitian of the nature of the dissease and remedy. A Physitian is and should be an Imitatour of nature and an helper of nature. But how few have the Knowledge of the secret mysterys of physick? I have seen and read many authors, the best part of 30. Yet I never met but with one that did discover (explain) these mysterys plainly and to any good purpose. I cannot but admire the ignorance of the most practitioners that are many of them accounted brave, knowing men in those respects. But where God denys means and opportunity to know and improve, we must be silent. The using of Medicines in the gross substance without any separation of the Elements, pure part from impure part, the passive earth and the passive water that do no good but hinder, I shall now with God's leave declare what I understand in these mysterys as plainly [Page 220] and briefly as I can for the good of such as stand in need.

There is a thre[e] fold Substance in Vegitables, Minerals & Animals called Sal, Sulphur, Mercury.

To begin first with Vegitables. They are separated by Distillation & calcination. Thus first distill a plant or herb (being in the prime, that is, when it is sodded) in a Limbec. The oyl that swims upon the top of this water is the Sulphur. The water that hath the tast of the plant is the mercurial part.[147] The herbs remaining in the still must be burnt to Ashes. Every one of these must be kept a part, that is, the oyl from the water, and the water from the oyl, in vessels close stopt a part.

Then take the ashes of the distilled herbs or the Ashes of the same sort of herbs that were not distilled for that yeilds salt; the distilled herbes, very little. Take these Ashes a quantity and steep them in warm water 3 or 4 days & stir them up 3 or 4 times a day. Clear off through a Hippocras bag. Filtre it with Tongues or shreds [of fabric]

146. That is, the patient will desert one physician at the request of another.
147. Cf. p. 218.

till it be as clear as running *water*, and then boyl up this liquour to a salt. Dissolve it in water and boyl it up again, then it is clear. The oftner so done, the better. This is called the fixed salt.

Then take this salt & dissolve it in the distilled water of the same herb (having the tast of the herb).[148] Let it be kept warm for 48 hours, then vapour away (boil off) the liquour or distill it, and the fixed salt will have drawn the strength of the water to it, or the Volatile salt so called, and so encreased in quantity.[149]

Keep it in a glass and the oyl of the plant called the sulphur with it. Let them stand together till they be mixed or become a body, and that will be in half a year's space. Add spirit of wine to it. A few drops of this medicine is enough for anybody. [Page 221]

This is called a Quintessence, and Elixear in the Balsamic medicine. It may seem incredible that a writer speake of this medicine so prepared. For my own part it is the best preparation of medicine that is or can be made. For I know by experience no medicine like a fixed vegitable salt [to] so cleanse a sore and make it have laudable quitter. And for easing of pain inward and outward, nothing like Vegitable Sulphur or oyl for refreshing the faint body. These in a body together must never be better than either or them used alone by it self. [Page 222]

An Excellent Medicine out of Distilled Salt Peter as followeth.

Take Salt peter one or 2 pound. Distill it in a glass Alembic in sand as if you would distill aqua fortis. Put fire under it and moderate the same by degrees. Encrease it 3 or 4 hours after the fire. Continue in the highest degree 5 or 6 hours and then thou shalt see the Spirits of saltpeter have penetrated the glass. Take it off with a soft fether on the out side. It showeth all sorts of colours lively. That [which] is in the bottome is white as snow and wholly fined. Its a remedy to extinguish all fevers, the dose from ½ dram to 1 dram. Dissolve in some component liquour. This Remedy hath not the like to cut and

148. What Palmer calls the mercurial or volatile salt.
149. That is, the fixed and the volatile salts will now be combined.

cleanse & purge, to evacuate corruption of humours, to preserve the body from all pollution of corruption. It is [of] the nature of balsamic salt and must needs have the vertues. The spirit of saltpeter is sour and tart & wonderfull cold.

Observation. When Salt Peter is made there is a marine salt extracted out of the liquour the salt peter is congealed in. See how to make salt peter in the latter end of the book.

Take the Salt Peter and the marine salt either apart or both together. Put into a retort with a receiver. With the fire heat comes a sharp sour salt, mercurial. Then with a greater heat a salt sulphurous, nitrus sweet. The third salt is fixed and will not [vaporize] with fire. What these will doe when they are fixed together, he is a phylosopher that knows and improves.

Note that Salt peter is the special Key & cheife porter (agent) that openeth most hard bodys and the most sollid things, as well stones as mettalls, and bringeth (dissolves) Gold and Silver into liquour with the proper waters, extracted out of the whole mass without seperation of the [illegible] or fixed. And as it makes all bodys metallic, spirited (gaseous), and volatile, so on the contrary part it hath worked to fix and incorporate spirits, how flying so ever they be.[150]

Vid. Pag. 231 of the sp. of s.p. [saltpeter] & how to make S.P. [Page 223]

Culpepers Antidote for paines of the brest, sides, belly by wind & stitches, to remove the paine of the Liver by opening of obstructions, of Reins and Kidneys by provoking of Urine.[151]

Rx. Nitre, Pepper, Cumin Seeds, of all alike; as much Rue as the weight of all the rest. Make it into an Electuary with hony. John Gerard speaks of this in verse in the Vertues of Rue.[152] The dose is not described. If you add powder of Calamus, I suppose it will be the better, or gentian or bay berrys, aristolochia rotund[a], all or any of them, add to the former ingredients.[153] [Page 224]

150. No matter how volatile they are.
151. This prescription could not be found in the *Pharmacopoeia*.
152. Gerarde does devote a full page (1633, p. 1257) to the virtues of rue, but not in verse.
153. An example of pharmacological reasoning of this period. Of simples considered to help specific complaints, any or all of them might be combined to advantage.

Tansy

Saith Culpeper, the reason why men are so sickly in the summer is because that they eat not good store of Tansy in the spring. It consumes coald and phlegmatick humours. The infusion in wine or juice in wine a remedy for all diseases that come of stopping of urine, strangury, good for wind in stomach, belly, matrix, it carries humours downward that trouble the stomach, keeps from abortion. Vid. Eng. Physit.[154]

Wild Tansy

For all fluxes of blood in men or women. Pouder of the dry herb & coral & ivory; mix together and taken in the distilled water of the herb steeped & applyd to the soals of the feet & wrists doth abate hott fitts of agues be they never so violent.

Preserved Enula Campana

For shortnes of breth, cough, spitting blood, pain of the sides, strengthen the stomach & digestion, cleanse from all unclean humours the stomach, breake the stone, move the terms, heale ulcers of all the inward parts.

Conserve of Betony

For cramp, palsy, Epilepsy, madnes, spitting of blood, paine of bladder, Kidnys, liver, melt (milt), for Dropsy, against all venom and all inward sickness

Conserve of Borrage or bugloss

For all venom & pestilential agues, strengthen the heart and vital spirits, cleanse the blood of all melancholly, coole all inward parts. This conserve is *made* of the blew flowers.

154. A reference to Nicholas Culpeper's *The English Physitian* (1652), pp. 367–68.

Conserve of Fumitory

Against venomous air, cleanseth the blood corruptions, openeth the liver and all inward parts, drives out the yellow jaundice by urine. It expelleth bad humours by sweat. This Conserve should be made of the flowers. The dose the quantity of a great nut at a time. [Page 225]

Preserved Calamus

Is like to Ginger in all his force. For all weaknes of the stomach, by reason of cold humours. Taken in the morning, preserves from all pestilential air. Its good for disseases of the bladder & kidnys, for stone, gravel, womens terms. Opens all obstructions.

Preserved Berberrys

For the bloody flux. Cools the blood heated by choller, it obstructeth womens Courses or terms, makes appetite. To meat it hath the nature of Conserve of Roses, yet something stronger. This should be bathed in wine and boyld with sugar after they are strained through a scarfe.

Conserve of Elder-Berrys

Against all inward venom, it cures all ulcers & swellings, it expelleth by sweat all bad humours. It is to be taken before one go to the bath, after purg[ing] and that fasting. If this be so used it doth consume the dropsy in the beginning. It hath been found that if this Conserve be spread upon the rose that thereby it will immediately wear away.[155]

Conserve of Elder Flowers

Opens the Liver, drives away the swellings of the belly, & beginnings of dropsy. [Pages 226–29 are missing. Page 230]

155. *Rose* here refers not to the flower but to the disease erysipelas.

Oyl of Elder-Flowers

Made as oyl of Camomile. With sallade oyl taketh away all pain of the joynts.

Oyl of Mint, so made

Warms a cold stomach, takes away vomiting, provokes appetite, helps Consumption, consumes all hard swellings.

Oyl of Water-lilly-Flowers

For them cannot rest [from] paine of Kidnys, of heat, against lust, annoint the privitys. It is of the nature of oyl of Violets, not so cold as oyl of Poppys.

Oyl of Wormwood

It strengtheneth the stomach & opens all the inward parts. [Applied] to the navil, kills worms, more profitable than wormseed, it is to be made with sallade oyl, and add half so much roses as wormwood. [Page 231]

This Spirit of Salt Peter is not hot in quality but rather cold as appears by the tart and sharp tast thereof, and is far different from the Elementary coldnes, for that it can dissolve bodys, and coagulate spirits, no less than it doth congeale salt peter, which sournes is the general cause of fermentation and coagulation of all natural things.

How to make Salt-Peter

Take fit (suitable) earth[156] and pour upon it common hot water as they make lye out of ashes.[157] Let it run through it. The water will be brackish. Boyl away two thirds. Let it stand and cool, and the salt peter will be on the top like Ice. Take it off, dissolve it in water

---

156. Unfortunately Palmer does not tell the reader how to find "fit" earth.
157. Lye was leached from wood ashes.

and purify it. The other water of the first separation, boyl it to a salt that will be like marine salt.[158] [Page 232 is blank. Page 233]

Tincture of Mars

Take filings,[159] 2 oz.; Tartar or Cream of Tartar, 6 oz. Boyl it in water in an Iron pott, so much water as will cover it, and keep it boyling 4 days together. Add sugar afterwards to the water to keep it from souring. Or when the water is boyled much away, add brandy or spirits of wine. This will keep. This is a better Balsam than can be made of herbs. It cures ould soars without quitter and skales the bone by turning the scale round in the soar. And healeth up the soar. There may also be made a Tincture of Coppar after the same manner for the same use, not safe to be used inwardly as the former may. [Page 234]

Diaphoretical Antimony

Calcine Antimony till it be very white, wash it in warm water often that it have no tast. Strain the water of[f], dry it. Take 10 grains in pap of apple to ease and take away great inward paine and procure sweat. [Page 235]

Oyl of Antimony

Rx. Crude Antimony and crude Tartar being powdred & close luted in a pott, no air can come in or breath forth. Set in a potters Furnace. By this it is made a past[e], blackish and swarthish, red of colour. This brought into a powder, putt into another pott well glased. On it pour distilled Vinagar [so] that it may lye two fingers breadth above. Set on a furnace to be heated. Let it stand on a furnace to be heated. Let it stand on a furnace for 3 or 4 hours. Still add more to it untill it have no more rednes in the Vinagar.

158. By this procedure the author expected to separate saltpeter, or potassium nitrate, and marine salt, or sodium chloride.
159. Iron filings. Mars was the god of iron.

Distill by a Limbic untill the red substance remaine in the bottom. Break the glass. Take the whole forth that sticketh to the glass and put it in a Hippocras bag made of white cloth. The same hang in a cellar where the oyl will distill by drops into a glass having been set under same. Set it 40 days in horse dung till it be an oyl. It easeth all paines of wounds, healeth them perfectly, troublesom cancred ulcers.

Or take Vinagar 3 times distilled with powder of Antimony as before. Set upon the embers till it become red by boyling. Doe it several times till the Vinagar draw off all the rednes. Distill them in a Retort luted [until] the first is clear. When the red drops appear, change the Receiver. Increase the fire till all be come forth.

This Quintessence of Antimony kept in a glass close stopped that no air breath forth is the miraculous oyl that mortifys all kind of wicked ulcers by bathing them with the said oyl. This healeth them in a short time with easines. The quantity of one drop given at a time by the mouth with wine or broth, or any other distilled water, doth as well empty the body by vomiting as downward by siege. And this given to a sick person doth thoroughly cure him of any crude or malignant kind of sicknes. As by a tryal a further truth may be known, *let but the practice* [be] learned. Note: it must be the sharpest Vinagar.[160] [Pages 236 and 237 are blank. Page 238.]

Pills

Saponaceous for Jaundice

Saponis Venet., 2 drams.
Rhubarb, 1 dram.
Syrop Croci sativ. to form 36 pills.
Dose four [pills].

Steel Pills

Limat. Ferri, 1 dram.
Ext. of gent. ochro, 1 dram.

---

160. The pages that follow are in several hands, probably as later owners made additions to blank pages. Page 245 is partly in Palmer's hand.

Make 24 [pills]. Dose, 4. Ter vel quater per diem.
Ferri vitriolat., 1 dram.
Ext. corticis, 1 dram.
Circa 24, dose 2. Ter vel quater in die. [Page 239]

Medicated Wine or Beer

Gentian
Lemon peel of each 4 oz.
[Illegible]
Bacc. Juniper 2 oz.
Cinnamon 2 oz.
Rubig a ferri 1 oz.

Hemlock plaister

Expressed juice of Hemlock 4 oz.
Gum ammoniac 8 oz.
Vinigear of Squills, sufficient to dissolve the juice. Add the juice
to the solution. Strain it and boil it to the consistence of a plaister. [Page 240]

Mercurial girdle

Hydrargyrum, 3 drams, well shaken with Succ. Limon, 2 oz., till
the globules cease to appear. Pour of[f] the liquor and to the killed
quicksilver add half the yolk of an egg, 1 scruple [of] gum tragacanth,
finely powdered. Spread this on a flannel roll 3 fingers breadth, long
[enough] to encircle the waist & there worn.[161] [Page 241 is blank.
Page 242]
Swellings [page] 55
Canker of throat 73
Burns
Pills, jaundice 238 [Page 243 is blank. Page 244]

161. The mercurial girdle was considered antisyphilitic and useful in treating skin
diseases.

Of Phlebotomy and Admin[istering] Physick

In Youth let blood from the change [of the moon] to the first quarter. In middle age from the first Quarter to the Full. In elder years from the Full to the last quarter. In old age from the last Quarter to the Change.[162] But under the age of 14 and over the age of 56 it is not good to bleed at all. Again in Dog-dayes it is very hurtfull to take Physick at all unless there be great need. In such a case the Disease being desperate, the cure must be adventured.

Purge when the Moon is in one of these Signs, Cancer, Scorpio or Pisces & it will be sure to work the better, for in a moist sign the humours of the body are then stirred up and down & the better purge out. In this case it cannot be amiss to prepare humours by something that's laxative. Let this be done when the Moon is either in Gemini, Libra or Aquarius.

Take a Vomit that it may work thoroughly when the Moon is in Aries, Taurus or Capricorn.

And in letting of blood as aforesaid, Beware the sign lie not in that part of the body which is let blood, but rather at a considerable distance therefrom.[163]

Vide Pag. 15 of the Nature of the 12 Signs of the Zodiack.[164] [Page 245, partly in Palmer's hand.]

Cor ardet, Pulmo loquitur, Fel commovet Iras, Splen ridere facit, cogit amare Iecur.

i.e., The Heart doth burn, the Lungs do speak,

The Gaul to Ire doth move;

The Spleen or Milt doth make us laugh,

The Liver makes us love.

Mizaldus[165]

---

162. Note how the age-groups for phlebotomy are correlated with the age of the moon.

163. Astrological theory held that each part of the body was under the influence of a particular planet.

164. This book is not further identified.

165. Antoine Mizauld, or Mizaldus, was a French physician and mathematician and the author of many works on medicine, astrology, and gardening. He died in

Elizabeth Palmer my dear Mother died the first day of February Anno Dom. 1687/8[166] in the 45th year of her age. She *would have been* 45 *if she had lived till the middle of February.*

Thomas Palmer my dear Father deceased at Port royal in Jamaica June the 16, 1689 *aged forty* 50 years.[167]

Elizabeth Palmer my dear Mother deceas'd April 16, 1740. Aged about 64.

June 17, 1743. My dear Father Thomas Palmer deceas'd in the 78th year of his Age.

Tu Deus O Mentem da sanam in Corpore sano! Hic placidum ut Vitam vivamus ibique beatam.[168]

1578. His verses quaintly summarize a theory of the control of the emotions by the various bodily organs.

166. By our reckoning this would be 1688. This Elizabeth was the author's mother.

167. Evidently there was uncertainty as to when the author's father was born, as the ages at death stated in shorthand and clear hand do not agree.

168. Thou, O Lord, give us a healthy mind in a healthy body. Here may we live a peaceful and so a blessed life.

Glossary

The actions of the remedies listed below are those reported by writers of past centuries. The actual effects of the drugs may or may not be as described. The author takes no responsibility for the safety or efficacy of any substance or mixture listed here or elsewhere in this book. Some of them may even be dangerous. The interested reader is advised to consult a modern textbook of pharmacology.

All quotations are from the 1675 edition of Culpeper's *Pharmacopoeia Londinensis*.

The catchwords, some misspelled, are as Palmer wrote them.

abstersive. Detergent.
aceto dissolutum. Dissolved in vinegar.
acetum nilliticum. Probably *Acetum scillicum*, vinegar of squills.
Achillea millefolium. Common yarrow, once used in treating wounds.
acorus, *Acorus calamus*, sweet flag.
ad tophas dissolvendo. For dissolving tophi, concretions found in gout.
agaric. The fungus *Boletus*. Cathartic, emetic, antidiaphoretic.
Agaricus albus. See *agaric*.
Agnus castus. A variety of *Verbena*. Antaphrodisiac.
agrimony. *Agrimonia*, cocklebur. Astringent.
ague. Intermittent fever, chills.
albugo. Leucoma, a white opacity of the cornea.
album graecum. White dung of a dog.
alchornes. *Alchornea latifolia*, alcornoque, a South American tree. Its bark was tonic and astringent.
alembic. A still.
alexipharmic. A remedy defensive against poison, sickness.
alia. Others, e.g., other remedies.
alicampane. *Elecampane, q.v.*

aliud. Another, e.g., another remedy.

alkermes. A cordial. Culpeper quotes the College of Physicians' recipe:

"Take of the juyce of Apples, Damask-rose-water, of each a pound and a half: in which infuse for twenty four hours, raw silk four ounces strain it strongly, and add syrup of the berries of *Chermes* brought over to us, two pound: Sugar, one pound, boyl it to the thickness of Honey: then removing it from the fire whilst it is warm add Ambergreece cut small half an ounce, which being well mingled put in these things following in powder, Cinnamon, Wood of Aloes, of each six drams: Pearls prepared two drams, Leaf-Gold a dram, Musk a scruple, make it according to Art. . . . give not too much of it at a time, lest it prove too hot for the body, and too heavy for the purse" (pp. 158–59).

allchymilla. *Alchemilla*, a plant of the rose family. Astringent for hemorrhage.

allom. *Alum*, q.v.

almonds of the throat. Amygdala, tonsil.

almons down. Almond bloom, a liquid cosmetic of Brazil dust, water, isinglass, alum, borax, etc.

aloes. *Aloe barbadensis*. Cathartic, stimulant, emmenegogue, stomachic, anthelminthic.

aloes cicatrine. Probably *Aloe socotorina*. See *aloes*.

aloes F. Probably *Aloe ferox*.

aloes ros. *Aloes rosata*, aloes washed with rose juice.

alophangia. See *pilulae alaphangiae*.

Althaea. The mallow family. Emollient, demulcent.

alum. Potassium aluminum sulphate. Astringent.

amber-greise. Ambergris, a concretion from the intestine of the sperm whale.

ammoniacum. *Gummi ammoniacum*, resin from the juice of *Dorema ammoniacum* or *Ferula tingitana*. Expectorant, antispasmodic. Also used to make plasters.

ana. Of each.

anagallis. The plant red pimpernel. Stomachic, antispasmodic.

anasarca. See *oedematous*.

angelica. The stalk, leaves, and seeds were considered aromatic and carminative.

anodyne. A pain reliever.

anthelmintic. An agent to expel or destroy intestinal worms.

Anthos tunicis. *Rosmarinus*, rosemary. Given in wine or tea as a diuretic. Also for headaches, dyspepsia, sleeplessness.

antiloimic. A remedy against plague.

antimonii vitrum. Glass of antimony.

antimonium diaphoreticum. Antimony oxide. Emetic, cathartic, diaphoretic.

aperient. A gentle laxative.

apostem. Impostume, abscess.

apostume. See *apostem*.

apple. Pupil of the eye.

aq. *Aqua*, water.

aqu. colat. *Aqua colata*, filtered water.

aqu. cuscute et sucuere. Water of cuscuta and succory.

aqua angelica. A distillate of angelica, carduus, fennel, etc. Aromatic and carminative.

aqua asparag. *Aqua asparaga*. Probably an infusion of asparagus.

Aqua betonica. Extract of betony.

aqua carduus benedicta. Water of *Centaurium*, blessed thistle.

aqua celestis. A distillate of numerous ingredients.

aqua mulsa. Hydromel, q.v.

aqua pastoris bursae. Water of shepherd's purse.

aqua plantag. *Aqua plantaginis*, water of the plantain.

aqua rosae. Rose water.

aqua vitae. Alcohol, brandy.

arch-angel. *Angelica archangelica*. Carminative, diuretic.

argila cum aceto. Aluminum acetate.

Aristolochia rotunda. A variety of birthwort.

armoniack. See *ammoniacum*.

aromat. rosat. letific. Galeni. *Aromaticum rosatum laetificans Galeni*, an aromatic and cordial confection of roses.

aron. *Arum.* Many species. The roots were used in asthma, consumption, etc.

arsenicum. Arsenic.

arteria aspera. Trachea.

ascia. A fish, not further identified.

ascites. Hydrops, dropsy, accumulation of fluid in abdomen.

assafoetida. Extract of *Ferula asafetida.* Antispasmodic, stimulant, anthelmintic.

auripigmentum. Orpiment, arsenic trisulphide, a poisonous pigment. Once used as a depilatory.

available. Efficacious.

avens. A plant of the genus *Geum.* Used internally for indigestion and externally for wounds.

axonge. Axunge, axle grease.

bacc. Juniper. *Baccae juniperi,* juniper berries.

Baccharum lauri. "An herb used by the ancients . . . to destroy enchantment" (Dunglison). Identity uncertain.

balnea Maria. Marian bath, a kettle of water with straw in the bottom. See *Admirable Secrets,* p. 57.

balsam. Resin, benzoic acid, and sometimes an essential oil.

balsam of Lucatello. An ointment of wax, oil, turpentine, sherry, and balsam of Peru, colored with dragon's blood, q.v.

balsam of Peru. Resin of *Myroxylon Pereirae,* a tropical American tree.

balsam Samech. Distillate of wine combined with salt and oil.

balust. Balaustine flowers from *Punica granatum,* the pomegranate. Astringent.

barrow. A castrated young pig.

basilicon. Ointment of yellow wax, black pitch, resin, and olive oil.

batones. Probably betony, q.v.

bawm. Baume, balsam.

Bay salt. Coarse salt from seawater.

bdellium. Gum resin from *Myrrha imperfecta.*

bed ward. Toward bedtime.

belly ake root. *Angelica.* Aromatic, stomachic, tonic.

benedicta laxativa. See *confectio sennae.*

berberry. *Berberis*, the barberry bush.
Beta rubra. Red beet root.
betony. *Betonica officinalis*. An ancient remedy, little used later.
bever cod. Beaver scrotum.
bezoar. Concretion found in digestive tracts of animals. Antidote against poison.
binding. Constipating.
bizant. simpl. *Syrupus Byzantinus simplex*, q.v.
black hellebore. *Helleborus niger*. Cathartic.
bole. *Bolus*, mass.
bole Armoniack. Probably Armenian bole, a red clay. Styptic.
bombast. Cotton padding.
borage. *Anchusa officinalis*, bugloss, a blue-flowered plant. Aperient.
brake root. See *polypody*.
brank-ursine. *Acanthus mollis*, bear's breech. Mucilaginous and demulcent.
bray'd. Pounded.
Brazil dust. Sawdust from Brazil wood, *Caesalpina echinata*.
bresica. *Brassica*, a family including turnip, cabbage, rutabaga, cauliflower.
brimstone. Sulphur.
Bruscus. Wild myrtle, butcher's broom. Provokes urine, breaks stone.
bugloss. See *borage*.
burdoch. Burdock, *Articum lappa*. The roots are diuretic; the seeds, cathartic.
burnet. *Pimpinella*, an astringent and tonic plant.
bushel. A vessel holding a bushel.
by fitts. Intermittently.

calam. aromat. *Calamus (Acorus) aromaticus*, "sweet Garden Flag. It provokes Urine, strengthens the Lungs, helps bruises, resists poyson, & c." (Culpeper, 1675, p. 3).
calamint. *Clinopodium calamintha*. Was dried and sprinkled on excoriated surfaces.
calcine. To heat so as to drive off water or other liquids.
callome. *Callum*, hard skin.

calor naturalis. Natural heat.

calx viva. Quicklime.

camomile. *Anthemis.* The dried plant was a bitter tonic and stomachic. Used externally in fomentations.

camonomile. See *camomile.*

Cancer fluv. *Cancer fluviatilis,* river crab.

cantharides. Dried bodies of *Lytta,* Spanish or blister fly. Externally a vesicatory. Internally an intense genitourinary irritant.

caper. *Capparis,* a low, prickly shrub. Buds and fruit are used in condiments.

cardamom. Fruit of *Elettaria cardamomum.* Restorative.

card. ben. *Carduus benedictus,* blessed thistle. Emetic, diaphoretic, tonic.

Carduus. Thistle.

carminative. Causing expulsion of flatus.

Caryophilus. The pinks family. Stimulant, carminative.

Cassia. Large genus of the senna family.

caster distel. *Castor destillatum,* distilled castoreum, q.v.

castoreum. A skin secretion of the beaver.

castorium. See *castoreum.*

castor ungul. *Castoris ungula,* beaver's claw.

cataplasm. Poultice.

caul. Amniotic membrane. Also, omentum.

caustic. Corrosive substance used to break down dead tissue.

cautery. Hot iron used to destroy tissue or check hemorrhage.

celandine. *Chelidonium majus.* Emetic, cathartic, diuretic.

centaury. *Sabbatia angularis,* American centaury. Tonic, stomachic.

cephalea. *Cephalea hemicrania,* migraine.

cera alba. Bleached beeswax.

cera cum resina. Beeswax with resin.

cera resinae. See *cera cum resina.*

cerate. Mixture of wax, lard, or oil as base for an ointment.

ceratum santalinum. *Ceratum sandalinum,* salve of saunders, roses, bole Armenian, camphor, white wax, and oil of roses, all made into a plaster.

cere citrin. *Cera citrina,* citrus wax.

cerecloth. Cloth on which ointment is spread.

cerus. *Cera*, beeswax.

cerussa. Basic lead carbonate, white lead. Used in plasters.

cervi genitale exsiccatum & in pulvere redactum. Deer's genitals dried and powdered.

cesei veteris & acris. *Caseus vetus et acer*, old and sharp cheese.

ceterach. European scale fern.

chamomel. See *camomile*.

cherish. Warm.

chermes. Kermes, dried bodies of cochineal-like insect. Contains purplish dye.

chicory. *Cichorium*, succory. Tonic.

china. *Cinchona*. Bark was medicinal.

chin cough. Pertussis, whooping cough.

choler. Yellow bile, one of the four humors.

chyle. Food absorbed from intestine.

chymical. Chemical. Formed by chemistry, in contradistinction to *Galenical*.

Cicer. *Cicer arietinum*, the chick-pea.

cichory. Chicory, q.v.

cinamo electi. *Cinnamomum electum*, choice cinnamon.

Citrullus. *C. vulgaris*, watermelon.

clary. Clarified mixture of spices, wine, and honey.

cleonin. Uncertain, but perhaps the diaphoretic plant *Gynandropsis*.

clottered. Clotted.

clout. Cloth.

clovenswort. *Ranunculus*, clovewort, crowfoot. Counterirritant.

clown's wort. Clown's woundwort, *Stachys*. Vulnerary.

clyster. Enema.

cochia. Purgative pill.

cod. Scrotum.

cole, colewort. Cabbage.

colocynthis. *Citrullus colocynthis*, bitter apple. Cathartic.

colophony. Black residue from distilled turpentine.

colt's foot. *Asarum canadense*, Canada snakeroot, wild ginger. Stimulant, diaphoretic.

columella. Uvula.

comfrey. *Symphytum* roots. Emollient.

concoction. Digestion as understood in the seventeenth century.

condit. *Conditum*, compound of wine, honey, and aromatics.

confect. Alchorines. *Confectio Alcornea*. See *Alchornes*.

confection. Anything preserved or made with sugar.

confection of Alkermes. Syrup of apple juice, damask rose water, syrup of chermes, sugar, ambergris, cinnamon, wood of aloes, pearls, leaf gold, musk. Stimulant.

confectio sennae. Senna, tamarind, cassia, prunes, coriander seed, liquorice, sugar, water. Laxative.

Conium. Poison hemlock.

Consolida major. Comfrey, q.v.

contra rupturam. Against rupture.

copperas. Copper sulphate.

coq. in aqua colat. *Coquata in aqua collata*, cooked together in water.

coquantur ad tertiam. Cooked to one-third.

coquin. Probably *coquinata*, cooked.

cordial flours. Flowers used to make a cordial.

cornu cervini usti. *Cornu cervi usti*, burnt deer's horn, hartshorn.

corrected. Made to taste less unpleasant.

cortex citri condit. Prepared citron peel.

costive. Constipated.

costmary. *Tanacetum vulgare*, tansy. Stimulant, diaphoretic.

couch grass. *Agropyron repens*, a weed. Used in urinary tract disorders.

counterirritation. Irritation induced, as in blistering, to relieve pain or disease.

courses. Menses.

cranbill. Probably crane's bill, *Geranium maculatum*. Astringent.

cranum human usto. *Cranium humanum ustum*, burned human skull. Antiepileptic, alexipharmic.

crocus martis. *C.m. adstringens*, colcothar, red iron oxide; *c.m. aperiens*, iron carbonate.

crocus metallorum. Sodium or potassium thioantimonite.

crop. Sprout, head of flower or herb.

crowfoot. *Ranunculus*. The roots would draw poison from a plague sore.

cucumber. *Cucumis*, q.v.

Cucumis. *C. sativus*, cucumber. Purged phlegm.

cucurbita. Gourd.

cum aqua pastoris bursae & plantaginis. With water of shepherd's purse and plantain, q.v.

cumarin. *Dipterix odorata*. The bean has a strong vanilla-like odor.

cummin. *Cuminum cyminum*, an Eastern plant with aromatic seeds.

cupping. Application to the skin of a heated vessel in order to raise a blister or promote bleeding.

cuscuta. Dodder, windweed, a parasitic plant with a strong odor.

cynoglossum. Hound's tongue. Aromatic, mucilaginous.

cypris roots. Roots of *Cyperus*, sedge.

dead palsy. Paralysis.

decoction. Boiling ingredients in fluid to extract soluble materials; also the extract itself.

decumbiture. Taking to one's bed when ill.

defensive. Substance applied to diseased area for protection from air, etc.

dehiscent. Agent that opens a closed wound.

deliquium. Something dissolved by taking up moisture from the air.

de minis. Probably for *de minimis*, at the least.

demulcent. Soothing.

deobstruent. Remedy used to remove an obstruction.

despumat. *Despumata*, with the froth removed, clarified.

despumed. See *despumat*.

diacalaminth. Powder of calaminth, pennyroyal, origanum, parsley, hartwort, and seeds of smallage, thyme, lovage, black pepper. Removes phlegm, provokes urine and menses.

diacalcytheos. Plaster of hog's grease, olive oil, gold litharge, omphacine, white vitriol, plantain water.

diacathamum. Probably *diacarthamum*, an electuary.

diacatholicon. Complex mixture of cassia, senna, etc. Cathartic.

diachilon compound. Plaster with fourteen ingredients.

diachilon magnum. A plaster of seventeen ingredients, including birdlime, oil of sheep's foot, and yellow wax. Dissolves inflammations.

diachilon simple. Made of linseed oil, fenugreek seed, marshmallow roots, old oil, and gold litharge.

diaciminum. Probably *electuarium dyaciminum*, composed mostly of spices.

diacodium. Red poppy flowers steeped in sugar water. Anodyne.

diacorum. An electuary of numerous spices, chick-peas, pine nuts, and sweet flag. For coughs, catarrh.

diagrydium. *Convolvulus scammonia*, scammony. Cathartic.

diaireos. Confection of *Iris*. Cathartic.

dialthea. See *ung. dialthea*.

diamargariton. Confection of pearls.

diamoron. Juice of unripe mulberries and blackberries boiled with honey. For sore mouths.

dianucum. *Mel nuceum*, honey of nuts. Juice of shells of green walnuts, gathered in the dog days and boiled with honey.

diapalma. Plaster of litharge, olive oil, zinc sulphate, etc.

diaphoenicon. Electuary made with dates.

diaphoretic. Causing perspiration.

diascordium. Complex electuary containing opium. For diarrhea.

diatessaron. Electuary of gentian roots, aristolochia, bayberries, juniper extract, and honey.

dictamnus. *Fraxinella*, a Eurasian plant. Emmenagogue, anthelminthic.

discusses. Dispels.

disenabled. Prevented.

dispatch. Complete, finish.

distel. *Destillatum*, distilled.

distemper. Disease.

diuretic. Stimulating production of urine.

dodder. *Cuscuta*, q.v.

dog days. Period between early July and early September.

dolor. Pain.

doubtless. Safe, reliable.

dragon's blood. Juice of *Calamus* or *Pterocarpus*. Astringent.

dragon water. Liquid from herb *Dracunculus*.

Egyptiacum. A preparation of vinegar, honey, and verdigris.

elecampane. The plant *Inula helenium*, "hot and dry in the third degree, wholsom for the stomach" (p. 6).

elect. caricostinum. Not identified.

electuary. Compounded of honey, syrup, and various powders, pulps, and extracts.

elixir. An alcoholic solution of medicines. See *quintessence*.

elixir proprietatis. Tincture of aloes.

emmenagogue. Producing the menses.

emollient. A substance to relax and soften inflamed areas.

emplastrum. Adhesive plaster.

emplastrum ad herniam. A complex plaster for hernia, kidney disease, abortion, etc.

emplastrum contra rupturam. Probably same as *emplastrum ad herniam*, q.v.

emplastrum de baccis lauri. Plaster of bayberries. Included also frankincense, mastic, myrrh, honey. To relieve pain, colic, wind.

emplastrum de meliloto. Contained melilot flowers, *Trifolium melilotus*, fenugreek, bayberries, wormwood, marjoram, etc. Eases melancholy, anodyne.

emplastrum diacalcitheos. See *diacalcytheos*.

emplastrum e cymino. Plaster of cummin seeds, bayberries, wax, rosin, and oil of dill.

emplastrum epispasticum. A blistering plaster.

emplastrum hystericum. Applied to the navel to treat "fits of the mother," or uterus.

emplastrum oxycroceum. Included saffron, pitch, colophony, yellow wax, turpentine, galbanum, gum ammoniac, myrhh, olibanum, and mastic.

emplastrum sticticum. Had thirteen ingredients.

emulcent. Makes an emulsion.

enteric. Enteritis, intestinal inflammation.

Enula. See elecampane.

epithime. Topical application but not an ointment or plaster.

erebinthum. *Acer*, a variety of maple tree. Bark was medicinal.

ering. Perhaps eryngo, *Eryngium maritimum*, sea holly. Aphrodisiac.

eskar. Eschar, a scab, crust, or slough.

euphorbium. *Euphorbia*, spurge. Astringent.

excoriate. To remove skin, as in an abrasion.

ex gr. *Exempli gratia, e.g.*, for example.

ext. corticis. *Extractum corticis*, extract of bark. Often in reference to cinchona bark.

eyebright. *Euphrasia officinalis*. For eye diseases.

falling of the fundament. Anal prolapse.

farina fabarum, hordeorum, et erebinthi. Meal of beans, barley, and maple bark.

f. *Fiat*, make.

F. catapl. *Fiat cataplasma*, make a poultice.

f. cerat. *Fiat ceratum*, make a plaster.

f. elect. *Fiat electuarium*, make an electuary.

f. empl. *Fiat emplastrum*, make a plaster.

f. pilul. *Fiat pilula*, make a pill.

f. potio. *Fiat potio*, make a potion.

f. pulvis. *Fiat pulvis*, make a powder.

f. ungt. *Fiat unguentum*, make an ointment.

featherfew. Feverfew, *Matricaria*. The flowers were tonic and stomachic.

fenugreek. *Trigonella foenum*. Used in poultices.

ferment. Heat.

ferri vitriolat. *Ferrum vitriolatum*, iron sulphate.

fetherfew. See *featherfew*.

fined. Purified.

first and last. On awakening and going to bed.

fistulo. Fistula, an abnormal passage between organs, from an organ to the skin, etc.

fleet milk. Skimmed milk.

flos sulphuris. Flower of sulphur, obtained by sublimation, q.v.

flos unguent. Not identified.
flours. Flowers; also menses.
flower de luce. *Iris*. Cathartic.
fomentary. A heating poultice.
fomentation. Application of a hot compress, sometimes medicated.
fontinal. Fontanelle, an artificial opening for discharge of a secretion.
four great cooling seeds. Seeds of *Cucurbita, Cucumis, Melo,* and *Citrullus*, q.v.
foveatur locus vesicae. Let the bladder area be warmed.
French barley. Milled barley.
fry. Burn, as by the sun.
fumitory. *Fumaria officinalis*. Emmenagogue, anthelmintic.

gad. A metal spike.
galanga. Galingale, *Alpina officinarum*. The root is stimulant, aromatic, antirheumatic.
galbanum. Extracted from *Bubon galbanum*, wild celery. Antispasmodic, expectorant.
gall. Bile.
gallop. Boil.
galls. Probably oak galls, bark growths produced by insects, etc. Powerful astringent.
gamboge. Orange-red resin from *Garcinia* tree. Emetic, cathartic.
Gargarion. Uvula.
gargarism. Gargle.
garlick. Garlic, *Allium sativum*. "It is hot and dry in the fourth degree, binds naughty and corrupt blood, yet is an enemy to all Poysons" (p. 1).
gaul. See *gall, galls*.
genista. Woad-waxen, a spring shrub. A diuretic, used in dropsy.
gent. ochro. *Gentiana*, snakeroot, one of many plants believed to cure snakebite.
germander. *Teucrium*, a small perennial shrub. Formerly applied to wounds.
greater cooling seeds. See *four great cooling seeds*.
green sickness. Chlorosis, a disease of young girls.

ground ivy. *Glecoma hederacea.* Expectorant and tonic.

groundsel. *Senecio vulgaris*, a herb. Refrigerant, antiscorbutic.

guaiacum. The resin and wood of *G. officinale.* Stimulant, purgative, diaphoretic.

guajacum. See *guiacum.*

gum ammoniac. Resin of *Ferula.*

gum Arabic. Gum of *Acacia senegal.*

gum carann. *Gumma caranna*, from the caranna tree. Used in plasters.

gum lacca. Purified secretion of a scale insect. Tonic, astringent.

gum mastic. See *mastic.*

gum tacamahaca. A fragrant resin from various tropical trees including *Protium* and *Calophyllum.*

gum tragacanth. Juice of *Astragalus gummifer.* Demulcent.

guttae. Drops.

gutta gambo. Gamboge, q.v.

hand. Hand's breadth, four inches.

handy. Manual.

hartshorn. Spirits of ammonia.

hectic fever. A recurrent, daily fever. Often occurs in tuberculosis.

helebore. Various species of the plant *Helleborus.* Antispasmodic, cathartic; poisonous in overdose.

hemicrane. *Hemicrania*, migraine.

hemlock. *Conium maculatum*, poison hemlock. Narcotic; poisonous in overdose.

henbane. *Hyoscyamus.* Narcotic, anodyne, antispasmodic.

hermodact. *Hermodactylus* root. Cathartic.

hicket. Hiccup.

hiera. Any of several electuaries.

hiera logadii. A mixture with thirty-two ingredients for melancholy, vertigo, convulsions, leprosy, etc.

hiera pachii. A purging confection.

hiera picra. Holy bitters, which contained *Aloes socotorina* and *Canella alba.*

hiera simple. See *hiera picra.*

hippocras bag. Hippocras, an aromatic, heavily spiced wine, was strained through a linen bag. Sometimes called a hippocras sleeve or Hippocrates' sleeve.

horse tail. *Equisetum*. Astringent.

housleek. *Sempervivum tectorum*. Leaves were applied to bruises, ulcers.

huckle. Hip.

humidum radicale. A liquid thought to give flexibility to the tissues.

humour. Blood, phlegm, yellow bile, or black bile.

hydrargyrum. Mercury.

hydronick. Watery.

hydrops. See *ascites*.

hypochondrea. *Hypochondrium*, the area of the upper and lateral abdomen.

hypostatical. Related to sediment or deposit.

hyssop wine. Chief ingredient was *Hyssopus officinalis*. Purgative, emetic, diuretic.

iliaca passio. *Iliac passion*, *ileus*, intestinal obstruction.

impostume. Apostume, abscess.

incarnative. Medicine thought to promote regeneration of flesh.

in carne suille salso. In salted hog's flesh.

incidant palsy. Incident, or falling palsy, i.e., epilepsy.

Indian bean. *Catalpa* pods. A decoction was used in asthma.

indurate. Hard, as inflamed tissue.

intingitur. It is dipped into.

inveterate. Chronic.

irees. Perhaps the plant *Iris*. Roots were astringent, cathartic, diuretic.

isop. Hyssop. See *hyssop wine*.

issue. A *fonticulus* or small ulcer produced by caustic or knife. A dried pea or seton was inserted so that the sore would continue to drain.

jalap. Extract of root of *Exogonium purga*. Purgative.

juglans. Bark of the white walnut, *Juglans cinerea*. Laxative.

jujube. Sweet fruit of *Zizyphus*.

julep. A sweet drink.

key. A samara, a one-seeded, winged fruit of the maple, elm, or ash.

killed. Mercury which has lost its fluidity through mixing with lemon juice or turpentine.

king's evil. Scrofula, tuberculosis of the lymph nodes of the neck.

knot gout. Perhaps gout in which chalky deposits appear under the skin.

knot grass. *Polygonum*, bindweed.

kye. Cattle.

lac sulphuris. Milk of sulphur, precipitated sulphur.

lapis calaminaris. Impure zinc carbonate.

lapis haematites. Bloodstone. Antihemorrhagic.

lask. Diarrhea.

laudanum opiatum. Aqueous extract of opium.

laudatum valde. Greatly praised.

launch. Lance, incise.

leanne. Leanness, emaciation.

lees. Dregs, sediment.

lenitive. Gentle.

lettuce. *Lactuca*, lettuce opium. Narcotic.

levisticum. See *lovage*.

lib. *Liber*, pound.

lib. q. s. *Libri quantum sufficiat*, as many pounds as necessary.

lignum aloes. Wood of aloes, q.v.

lignum coryli laudatum valde. The greatly praised wood of the hazelnut tree.

lignum vitae. See *guaiacum*.

limat. ferri. *Ferri limatura*, iron filings.

limbec. Alembic, q.v.

linctus. Cough syrup.

linimentum gummi elemi. Liniment of gum elimi, a fragrant resin of various tropical trees.

liquescat. Let it melt.

liquor of tartar. Solution of tartar.

list. Band or strip of cloth.

litharge. Lead oxide, white lead.

lithontriptic. A substance believed to dissolve urinary calculi or stones.

lixivium. A solution of lye.

lixivium mitioris. A mild lixivium.

loadstone. Magnetite, magnetic iron ore.

Lond. treacle. London treacle, *Theriaca Londinensis*, a poultice of cummin seed, bayberries, germander, etc.

long pepper of ginger. Possibly ginger root.

looch de pino. A lohoch or cough syrup of pine nuts and thirteen other ingredients.

looch de pulmone vulpis. Cough syrup of fox lung, liquorice, maiden hair, anise seed, fennel seed, sugar, coltsfoot, scabious water.

looch sanum. A cough syrup with twenty-three ingredients.

lovage. The plant *Levisticum*. Carminative, stimulant.

luci mandibula. Jaw of a pike, *Esox lucius*.

lunary tribute. Menstruation.

lupin peas. Seeds of *Lupinus*. Used in a poultice.

luted. Sealed.

m. morning.

madder. *Rubia*. Detergent, diuretic.

magestery of perls and corrall. Made from pearls and coral, ground and dissolved in vinegar. Liquor of tartar was added to the filtrate until a precipitate, the magistery, was formed.

maiden hair. *Adiantum pedatum*, a fern.

mallalote. *Trifolium*. See *melilot*.

mallow. *Malva*. Demulcent.

malmsey. Sweet, rich, aromatic wine.

m. & e. Morning and evening.

mandragora. Mandrake. Narcotic, cathartic.

manna. Condensed juice of *Fraxinus ornus*, a tree. Laxative.

marjoram. Origanum, q.v.

mars-mallows. Marshmallows, *Althea officinalis*. Emollient, demulcent.

mass. Paste.

mastic. Resin of *Pistacia lentiscus*. For dyspepsia, dysentery, gout.

mastichatory. Masticatory, a medicine to be chewed.

matrix. Uterus.

maudlin. *Chrysanthemum leucanthemum*, ox-eye daisy, maudlin wort. Antispasmodic, diuretic.

maw. Stomach.

may weed or pis-a-bed. Any of various diuretic plants.

mead. Fermented honey and water.

mechoacan. *Cypripedium*, moccasin flower, lady slipper. Used in nervous diseases.

medicated wine. *Vinum medicinale*, wine containing medicines.

megrim. Migraine.

melancholy. Black bile.

melilot. *Melilotus alba*, sweet clover. Used in fomentations, clysters; cathartic, expectorant.

melo. Melon.

mel rosarum. Honey of roses, alcoholic extract of roses with honey.

mel rosati. See *mel rosarum*.

mercury. The herb *Mercurialis*. Hypnotic, cathartic.

mezereo. *Daphne mezereum*, spurge olive. Bark is stimulant and diaphoretic.

milt. Spleen.

mirabolans. *Terminalia*, a dried Indian fruit. Laxative, astringent.

mirtles. *Vaccinium myrtillus*, myrtle berries.

misce; misceantur. Mix.

missenteary. Mesentery.

mithridate. A mixture with over twenty-five ingredients. Believed to expel poison.

mortify. To kill, as to mortify an ulcer.

mother. Uterus.

mother-time. Mother of thyme, *Satureja acinos*. Facilitated labor.

mould. The soft spot on the top of a baby's head.

mount royal. Not identified.

mouse ear. Various plants of *Pilosella*, *Hieracium*, or *Cerastium*.

mucilage. A mixture of mucus-like plant juices and gum.

mugwort. *Artemisia*, wormwood. Tonic, diuretic.

mullen. Mullein, the herb *Verbascum*. Demulcent, analgesic.

mumme. Dried human flesh.

munk's rubarb. Monk's rhubarb, *Rumex alpinus*. Purgative, blood purifier.

muscadine. Muscatel wine.

myrhh. Resin of *Commiphora*. Stimulant; used in asthma, bronchitis.

myrrha sarcocolla. Resin of *Penaea*. Astringent and detergent.

myrtus piperis. Probably *Myrtus pimenta*, pimento pepper. Stimulant, carminative.

napus. *Brassica*, the turnip.

nates. Buttocks.

navew. See *napus*.

neets foot oyl. Neat's foot oil, extracted by boiling cattle feet, bones, skin.

nep. *Nepeta*, catnip. Carminative, antispasmodic.

nerve oyl. *Unguentum nervinum*. An ointment with sixteen ingredients for nervous diseases.

nervine. A remedy acting on the nervous system.

nettles. *Urticaria*, useful in various diseases.

nigella. *Foeniculum*, fennel. Carminative, diuretic, antispasmodic.

nightshade. Either American *Solanum dulcamara*, blue nightshade, *S. nigrum*, black nightshade, or European *Atropa belladonna*, deadly nightshade.

nile tree. *Convolvulus*, morning glory. Cathartic.

nines. Perhaps "at nines," 9 A.M. and 9 P.M.

nitre. Potassium nitrate.

n. 8. *In numero 8*, eight in number.

n. x. *In numero X*, ten in number.

nux moschat. condit. *Nux moschatae condita*, prepared nutmeg.

nymphaea. Water lily. Demulcent, emollient.

occulus Indi. Possibly a corruption of *oculus mundi*, the opal.

oculus Christi. *Salvia*, wild clary. For diseases of eye, kidneys, etc.

oedematous. Swollen by fluid accumulated under the skin.

oil of almonds. Oil of *Amygdala dulcis* or *A. amarae*. Used for emulsions.

oil of bay. *Oleum laurinum*, from the laurel or bay tree.

oil of cestinum. Perhaps *oleum cicinum*, from *Ricinus communis*, the castor oil plant.

oil of nard. *Oleum nardinum* contained spikenard, aloes, marjoram, calamus, bay leaves, mace, oil of sesame, etc.

oil of Peter. Petroleum.

oil of tartar. Potassium subcarbonate that has taken up water.

oil of turpentine. Turpentine.

oil of vitriol. Sulphuric acid.

ointment of populeon. See *Unguentum populeum*.

ol. *Oleum*, oil.

ol. anisii. *Oleum anisi*, oil of anise.

ol. succini. *Oleum succini*, oil of amber. Stimulant, diaphoretic, rubefacient.

oleum amigd. dulc. *Oleum amygdalae dulcis*, oil of sweet almonds.

oleum camom. *Oleum camomili*, oil of camomile.

oleum capparib. *Oleum capparibus*, oil of capers, a complex mixture for diseases of the spleen.

oleum chym. absinth. Probably *oleum absinthi*, oil of wormwood.

oleum hyperici [et] terebinthi. Oil of Hypericon, q.v., white wine, earthworms, and turpentine.

oleum laurini. Oil of bay.

oleum lilioni. Oil of lily.

oleum rosae. Oil of damask rose.

oleum spicae. Oil of *Lavandula spica*, oil of spike.

oleum veteris. *Oleum vetus*, old oil.

oleum violae. Oil of violet.

olibanum. *Boswellia*, frankincense. Used in dysentery, etc.

omphacine. Verjuice, juice of sour grapes.

opening. Laxative.

opopanax. Gum resin from *Opopanax*. Antispasmodic, emmenagogue.

origanum. A genus of aromatic mints.

orris. Iris root.

oxicratum. See *oxycratum*.

oximel of squills. *Oximel scilliticum*, q.v.

oximel scilliticum. Oxymel of squill, *Scilla*.

oxycratum. Vinegar and water. Refrigerant, antiseptic.

oxycroceum. *Emplastrum oxycroceum*, a plaster of saffron, pitch, colophony, wax, etc.

oxymel. Honey and vinegar boiled to a syrup.

oyl of foxes. Made of fox fat, salt, dill, sage, rosemary, etc.

oyl of Hypericon. Infusion of *Hypericum perforatum*, St. John's wort, flowers in olive oil. Aromatic and astringent.

oyl of linnen rags. Perhaps linseed oil. Demulcent.

oyl of pepper. Oil of black and white peppers, myrobalans, smallage, fennel, oil of gilliflowers, etc.

oyl of sulphur. Sulphuric acid.

oyl of swallows. *Oleum hirundinum*, made with sixteen whole swallows and thirteen other ingredients.

papaver. Poppy, source of opium.

parietory. *Parietaria*, a wall plant. Diuretic, emollient.

passul. minor. *Passulae minores*, *Vitis corinthiaca*, currants. Cooling, stomachic.

peccant. Morbid, not healthy.

pellitory of Spain. *Anacyclus pyrethrum*, a sialogogue.

pellitory of the wall. See *parietory*.

peniroyal. Pennyroyal, *Mentha pulegium*. Oil was medicinal.

perfoliata. See *thorowax*.

philonium Romanum. Electuary of pepper, henbane, opium, and numerous other herbs in honey. Anodyne.

philupendula. Filipendula, *Spiraea filipendula*. Root was astringent, lithontriptic.

phlebotomy. Bloodletting.

phlegm. One of the four humors.

phrenzy. Frenzy.

p. i. *Per inde*, in the same manner as before.

picis nigri. *Pix nigra*, q.v.

pil. *Pilulae*, pills.

pil. sine quibus. Pills without which [I will not be]. Numerous ingredients. "It purgeth flegm, choler, and melancholy from the head, makes the sight and hearing good, and giveth ease to a burdened brain" (p. 186).

pill. asaserath. *Pilulae assaireth*. Hiera picra, mastic, citron, myrobalans, aloes, and syrup of stoechas. Purged choler and phlegm.

pills de tribus. See *pilulae de tribus*

pilulae alaphangia. Many ingredients. Cleansed stomach and brain of humors.

pilulae Arabicae. Made of aloes, briony, myrobalans, citron, and eleven other ingredients. For headache, vertigo.

pilulae arthriti. *Pilulae arthriticae.* For sore joints.

pilulae aureae. Golden pills. A complex mixture of herbs, seeds, etc. Anticarminative.

pilulae cochiae minor. Pills of aloes, scammony, syrup of wormwood, colocynthis, and purging thorn.

pilulae de agarico. Agaric and mumerous other simples. Cleared chest of phlegm.

pilulae de cochia fetida. See *pilulae foetidae.*

pilulae de cynagloss. Contained *Cynoglossum*, opium, myrhh, etc. For coughs.

pilulae de hermodactilis. A less violent purge than *pilulae foetidae*, which they resembled.

pilulae de hiera cum agarico. Pills of *hiera picra*, agaric, aloes, and honey of roses.

pilulae de iva. Presumably pills of *Teucrium iva.* See *germander.*

pilulae de sagapene. Pills of *Serapinum*, a kind of stinking gum.

pilulae de tribus. Pills of three things, a misnomer, since the ingredients were mastic, aloes, agaric, hiera picra, rhubarb, cinnamon, and syrup of succory.

pilulae foetidae. Stinking pills with nineteen ingredients. Purgative.

pilulae imperiales. Pills of aloes, rhubarb, agaric, senna, cinnamon, ginger, nutmeg, cloves, spikenard, mastic, and syrup of violets. Many virtues.

pilulae lucis majores. Contained thirty-seven ingredients. Eye remedy.

pilulae macri. They strengthen "both Stomach and Brain, especially the Nerves and Muscles" (p. 184).

pilulae mastichinae. Purgative pills of mastic, aloes, wormwood, agaric, hiera, and syrup of wormwood. Purgative.

pilulae pestilential. Presumably made from pestilential powder, which included seeds, herbs, pearls, sapphire, and bone of stag's heart.

pilulae Rudii. Purgative pills of aloes and colocynthis. "Keep your Chamber, they work very speedily, being of a penetrating nature."

pilulae Rufi. Pills of aloes and myrhh. Cleansing and strengthening.

pin and web. See *unguis oculi.*

pine nut. Seed of certain pines.

pinguid. Gal. veteris. *Pinguedo galli veteris,* fat of an old rooster.

piony. *Paeonia,* peony. The seeds "help . . . the fits of the Mother, and other such like infirmities of the Womb, stop the Terms, and help Convulsions" (p. 45).

pix liquida. Tar from *Pinus sylvestris.*

pix nigra. Black pitch.

pizel. Penis.

plantain. Any of various species of *Plantago.* Cooling, drying.

pneumatocele. An intrascrotal, gas-filled tumor or herniated length of intestine.

polypodium quercini. Polypody, q.v., growing on the oak tree.

polypody. *Polypodium,* bracken, brake root, a kind of fern.

pomegranate pills. Cool, bind, stay fluxes, help digestion.

pompholyx. Tutia, zinc oxide.

porrum. *Allium porrum,* the leek. Stimulating, diuretic.

posset. Milk curdled with acid, wine, or treacle; beer and milk.

postea adda. Afterward add.

powder of Ethiops. Mixture of tin filings, mercury, and sulphur. Anthelmintic.

prep. *Preparatum,* prepared.

presage. Prognostic sign.

presently. Promptly, at once.

pretious. Valuable.

probat. est. *Probatum est,* it has been tested (and approved).

pro renibus. For the kidneys.

proud. Excessive tissue, as in a healing wound.

prunella. The plant self-heal. Astringent; used in gargles.

pulv. Zeadoric. Powder of *Curcuma zedoaria.* The plant is a source of starch. Stimulant, carminative.

pulveris utriusque. Of each powder.

pulvis. Powder.

pulvis arsenicus. Apparently a powder of arsenious acid and mercury. Caustic.

pulvis arthriticus. See *Pil. arthriti.*

pulvis asphodelorum. Powder of *asphodel,* q.v.

pulvis bezoarticus Anglicus. Powder of English bezoar, q.v.

pulvis caryophilus. See *Caryophilus.*

pulvis consolid. major. Powder of *Consolida major,* symphite, q.v.

pulvis hermodact. *Pulvis hermodactylorum compositus,* powder of hermodactylus compound, a powerful purge. This plant was probably *Colchicum,* autumn crocus. "Take of men's bones burnt, Scammony, Hermodactyles, Turbith, Senna, Sugar, of each equal parts, beat them into a Powder . . . Dear Souls, avoid this Medicine, else the College [of Physicians] will have Men's bones enough to burn" (p. 153).

pulvis hydrargyrum. Powder of mercury.

pulvis testis apri. Powdered boar's testis.

purple grass. Red clover, spotted medic, or other plants with purplish flowers or foliage.

purples. Purpura, characterized by an eruption of purplish pustules.

purslane. *Portulaca oleracea.* Cold, dry.

putrid fever. Typhus.

pyrola. Wintergreen. Gentle astringent and tonic.

quartan. Recurring every fourth day.

quartern. A quarter of a pint, a gill.

quartile. In astrology, one-fourth of the circuit of the moon.

quick. Live, healthy.

quintessence. In medieval philosophy, the fifth essence; later, an alcoholic solution of a highly purified substance. See *elixir.*

q.s. *Quantum sufficiat,* as much as may be needed.

quitter. Pus, suppuration.

quotidian. Recurring daily.

radix Althea. *Radix Altheae,* root of Althea, q.v.

raisins of the sun. Sun-dried grapes.

rapontica. *Rheum rhaponticum,* rhubarb of Pontus. Perhaps the same as *R. officinale.*

rayne. Rein, kidney.

read betony. Red betony, probably wood betony, *Betonica officinalis.*

recepta. Prescription.

red saunders. Red sandalwood, *Pterocarpus santalinus*. See *dragon's blood*.

rein. Kidney.

renovetur 30 die. Let it be renewed on the thirtieth day.

requies Nicolais. *Requies Nicholaus*, a quieting electuary containing many substances including henbane, poppy, and mandrake.

resin pini. *Resina pini*, pine pitch.

resolution. Looseness, weakness.

restringent. Astringent.

retort. A vessel for distillation.

revulsion. To turn away a disease or poison from the affected part of the body.

rhabarb. electissimi. *Rhabarbari electissimi*, of the choicest rhubarb.

Rhenish. Rhine.

rheum. Any thin, watery discharge from mucous membranes; also rhubarb.

rhume. See *rheum*.

ribs. *Ribes*, a genus including blackberries, currants, gooseberries.

rock allom. Rock alum, a variety of ordinary alum.

roman wormwood. *Artemisia pontica*. Digestive, stimulant, anthelmintic.

rosa solis. *Narthecium*, bog asphodel; also the water made from the plant and many other ingredients.

rose. Erysipelas.

rosemary. *Rosmarinus officinalis*. Tops of plant are fragrant, aromatic. Diuretic; used also in liniment.

rowel. Seton, string, or other foreign object inserted under skin so that wound will stay open and drain, removing a humor.

rubia majoris. See *madder*.

rubig a ferri. *Robigo ferri*, iron rust.

rue. *Ruta*, herb of grace, "hot and dry in the third degree . . . helps difficulty of breathing, and inflammation of the Lungs . . . no herb resisteth poyson more" (p. 36).

ruscus. Wild myrtle, butcher's broom. Roots were aperient, diuretic.

sa., s.a. *Secundum artem*, according to art, in the usual way.

sabine. See *savin*.

sachar. *Saccharum*, sugar.

sack. Dry white wine.

saffron. *Crocus sativa* flowers. Stimulant, diaphoretic.

sagapen. *Sagapenum*, gum from *Ferula*, a genus yielding several medicinal resins. Antispasmodic, emmenagogue.

sage. *Salvia;* "hot and dry in the second and third degree, binding,
it stayes abortion" (p. 36).

Saint John's wort. *Hypericum.* Aromatic, astringent.

sal. Salt.

sal cum porro. Salt with garlic.

sal gemmae. Sodium chloride, table salt.

sal prunella. Saltpeter, potassium nitrate, fused into balls or sticks.

salat, salate. Salad.

sallot. Salad.

salt of angelica. Precipitate concentrated from a watery extract of the
bruised plant.

salt of tartar. Potash, potassium subcarbonate.

salt of wormwood. Wormwood ashes dissolved in water, filtered, and
evaporated to dryness.

salt rheum, salt rhume. Popular name for various eczematous and
herpetic diseases.

saltpeter. Potassium nitrate.

sambuci. *Sambucus niger*, elder tree. Cathartic.

samp. Coarse ground American Indian corn; porridge made from it.

sanguification. Making of blood; also transformation of venous to
arterial blood during respiration.

sanguis draconis. See *dragon's blood.*

sanicle. *Sanicula*, American herb used to treat intermittent fever.

saphene. Saphenous vein of foot and leg.

saponis Venet. *Sapo Venetiae*, Venetian soap. Similar to Castile soap.

sarcocolla. Resin from *Penaea sarcocolla*, an African shrub. Astringent, detergent.

sarsaparilla. Extract of root was mild tonic.

sassafras. Shrub or tree was stimulant, sudorific, diaphoretic.

sassaparilla. See *sarsaparilla.*

satyrium. *Goodyera pubescens*, scrofula weed, rattlesnake leaf, cancer

weed. An American Indian remedy; leaves were applied to scrofula sores.

saunders. See *red saunders*.

savin. Savin or sabine referred to both European shrub *Juniperus
sabina* and American red cedar, *J. virginiana*. Stimulant, emmen-
ogogue, abortifacient; externally irritating.

scabious. Various species of *Scabiosa*, once considered a remedy for
scabies.

scald head. A crusty or scaly disease of the scalp.

scammony. *Convolvulus scammonia*. Cathartic.

scarification. Making small incisions to draw blood.

schyrhus. Scirrhus, carcinoma.

scolopendria. *Asplenium*, spleenwort. Related to *ceterach*, q.v.
Mucilaginous.

scordium. *Teucrium scorodonia*, water germander. Tonic.

scorzonera. Viper's grass. Alexipharmic.

scouring. Flux, dysentery.

scrophularia. Figwort. Leaves and roots were remedy for scrofula,
warts.

scurf. Dandruff.

sea horse pizel. Penis of a walrus. Contains bone, the *os penis* or
baculum.

searse. To sift or strain.

sebestens. Fruit of *Sebestena*. Aperient.

seige. See *siege*.

sem. *Semen*, seed.

sem. agnus castus. Seeds of *Agnus castus*, q.v.

semina angelica. *Archangelica* seeds. Aromatic, carminative.

sempervivum. Houseleek. Emetic, cathartic, vesicant.

senna. *Cassia*. Laxative, diuretic.

sense. Sensation.

sephalus. Erysipelas.

seq. *Sequentes*, following.

seton. *Setaceum*, a twisted strip of linen or cotton placed in a wound
as a drain.

sextile. In astrology, one-sixth of the circuit of moon or planet.

sharp pointed dock. *Rumex*. For skin disorders.

shepheards grass. Probably *shepherd's pouch*, q.v.

shepherd's pouch. *Capsella bursa-pastoris*. Astringent.

shumach. Sumac, *Rhus*. Astringent, tonic.

sialogogue. Stimulates salivation.

sief album. Eyewash of sarcocolla, aloes, saffron, myrhh, boxthorn.

siege. Feces.

simpl. vel ex scillit. *Simplex vel ex scillitico*, plain or flavored with squill.

sincopis. *Brassica*, mustard.

singultus. Hiccup.

smallage. *Apium graveolens*, a variety of celery. Stomachic, diuretic, carminative.

small drink. Weak, nonalcoholic.

smith's water. Smithy water, *Ferraria aqua*, water from trough in which a smith quenched hot iron.

sod, sodden. Boiled, soaked, fermented.

solanum. Nightshade. Narcotic.

soldanella. *Convolvulus*, bindweed. Cathartic.

solomons seale. *Polygonatum*. Cathartic, diuretic, diaphoretic.

soluble. Gently relaxed bowels.

solutio diacatholicon. See *diacatholicon*.

solutive. Laxative.

sorrel. *Rumex*; "moderately cold and dry, binding, cutteth rough humors, cools the Brain, Liver, and stomach, cools the blood in Feavers, and provokes appetite" (pp. 16–17).

sothern wood. *Artemisia*. Aromatic.

spall. Brewers' term. Meaning unknown.

species. Mixture, compound powder.

species aromat. rosat. *Species aromatici rosati*, powder of aromatic roses.

species diaireos simplex. Orris root, sugar, *diatragacanthum frigidum*, made into powder. For chest diseases.

species diambre. Powder of cinnamon, angelica root, cloves, mace, nutmeg, galanga, cardamom, etc. Tonic.

species diamosch. See *species diamoses dulcis*.

species diamoses dulcis. A powder of eighteen ingredients including toasted raw silk, saffron, red corals, pearls, ginger, and musk. For melancholy, dizziness, palsies, etc.

species diarodon abbatis. The thirty-one ingredients included bone of stag's heart and red roses. Internally cooling.

species diatragacanthi frigidi. Gum tragacanth, gum arabic, starch, liquorice, various seeds, etc., made into an electuary. For chest diseases.

species elect. de gemmis. *Species electuari de gemmis frigidis*, a kind of electuary of cold jewels. Had eighteen ingredients including gold leaf, sapphire, emerald, ivory, and coral. Cordial.

sperage. Asparagus.

spermaceti. Whale oil.

spice nardi. Spikenard, *Aralia*. Aromatic.

spirit. Distillate.

spirit of sulphur per campanum. Sulphurous acid.

spirit of vitriol. Sulphuric acid.

spirit of wine. Alcohol.

spiritus vitr. *Spiritus vitrioli*, sulphuric acid.

sponge stone. Small, friable stone found in sponge. Lithontriptic.

spoonmeat. Liquid or semiliquid food fed with a spoon.

spruse. Spruce, *Picea*. Twigs and resin were used.

spuma argenti. Froth of silver, fused lead oxide.

spurge. See *euphorbium*.

s. q. Probably for *q.s.*, *quantum sufficiat*, q.v.

squill. *Scilla*. Root is emetic, purgative, diuretic, expectorant.

squinancy. *Cynanche tonsillaris*, quinsy, tonsillitis, or related inflammation.

staff seed. Seed of *Celastrus*, bittersweet, an American Indian remedy.

staves acre. Delphinium. Powdered seeds used to kill lice.

steeled wine. Contained iron salts.

steele pills. Contained an iron compound. See *steeled wine*.

stercus columbini [et] anatis. Droppings of pigeon and duck.

stibium. Antimony.

stiches. Stitches, sudden sharp pains.

stinking gladdon. *Iris foetidissima*, stinking iris. Narcotic, antispasmodic.

stomachic. Good for the stomach.

stone horse. Stallion.

stone pitch. Pitch of *Pinus sylvestris*, Scotch fir.

stoned. Having the seeds removed.

stones. Testes.

storax. A resin from *Styrax officinalis*. Stimulant, expectorant.

strait. Tightly constricted.

strangury. Difficult urination.

sublimate. Corrosive sublimate, bichloride of mercury. Very poisonous.

sublimation. Purification by transformation from solid to gas, then condensation to solid.

succ. limon. *Succus limoni*, lemon juice.

succini albi. *Succinum album*, white amber.

succum porri. *Succus porri*, garlic juice.

succus foedus. Filthy fluid.

succus glycyrr. *Succus glycrryhizae*, liquorice juice.

succus tabaccus. Tobacco juice.

sucori. Succory, chicory, *Cichorium intybus*.

suffer. Permit.

sulph. vivi. *Sulphur vivum*, native sulphur.

sumach. *Rhus*. Astringent, tonic.

summitatum antho. *Summitates Anthos*, tips of *Anthos*, q.v.

sup. Drink.

symphite. *Symphytum*, comfrey. Emollient.

syr. *Syrupus*, syrup.

syr. bugl. & de cort. citri. *Syrupus de buglosso & de corticum citroni*, syrup of bugloss and citron peel.

syr. de ros. sicc. *Syrupus rosae siccatae*, syrup of dried rose.

syr. of Cicory. *Syrupus de Chicorio*, complex infusion of chicory and many other herbs, made into syrup.

syr. of violets. Violets were steeped in boiling water, and sugar was added.

syr. of vitriol. Probably syrup of *Vitriola*, *Parietaria*, pellitory.

syr. ros. sol. *Syrupus rosarum solutivus*, solutive syrup of roses. Made with spring water, damask rose leaves, and sugar. "It looseth the belly, and gently bringeth forth choler and flegm, but leaves a binding quality behind it" (p. 129).

syr. tunicis. Syrup from the peels, e.g., citron peels.

syrop croci sativ. *Syrupus croci sativi,* syrup of crocus.

syrup acet. of citri. *Syrupus acitositatis citriorum,* syrup of lemon juice. Febrifuge, cooled the blood.

syrup of hyssop. Spring water, barley, smallage, parsley, fennel, liquorice, jujubes, sebestens, raisins, figs, dates, mallow seeds, quince seeds, gum tragacanth, hyssop, maidenhair, sugar. Cough remedy.

syrup of myrtles. Myrtle berries, red and white sanders, sumac, balaustine, barberry seeds, red roses, medlars, quince juice, pomegranates, sugar; "binding yet comforting" (p. 122).

syrup of poppies. See *Diacodium.*

syrup of stoechas. Lavender and rosemary flowers, perfumes, spices, etc. in syrup.

syrup. test of citri. *Syrupus testae citroni,* syrup of lemon peel.

syrupus Byzantinus simplex. Juice of endive and smallage leaves boiled with hops and bugloss. Helped yellow jaundice.

taccamahac. See *taecamahac.*

taecamahac. Tacamahac, resin of *Populus balsamifera,* a North American tree.

tamarisk. *Tamarix gallica.* Bark, wood, and leaves of this tree were medicinal.

tansy. *Tanacetum vulgare,* common tansy. Tonic, anthelmintic.

tartar. Potassium tartrate.

tenasmus. Tenesmus, painful spasm of anal sphincter and urgent desire to evacuate.

tent. Cylinder or roll of soft material used to keep a wound, sinus, or orifice open.

ter vel quater in die. Three or four in a day.

ter vel quater per diem. Three or four a day.

terebint. cocta. *Terebintha cocta,* refined turpentine.

terebinth. Turpentine.

terebinth Venetiae. Venetian turpentine, from *Pinus larix,* the larch.

terms. Menses.

terra sigillata rubia tincta. Red-colored sealed earth.

thapsia. *Thapsia asclepias*, Mediterranean herb. Vesicant and counterirritant.

theriac. Molasses containing opium. Also any of several remedies for venomous bites.

thorowax. *Bupleurum*. Aromatic, used in treating ruptures.

time. *Thymus*, thyme. Aromatic.

timpany. Tympany, tympanites, drumlike distention of abdomen with gas.

tincture. Alcoholic solution.

tincture of Mars. Alcohol, iron sulphate, and iron tartrate.

tongues. Tongs, slang for pantaloons or trousers. Hence, bags.

tophi. Calcareous particles in gouty joints.

topic. Locally applied.

tormentil. *Potentilla recta*. Root is astringent.

torrified. Heated.

tragacanth. See *gum tragacanth*.

transpiration. Perspiration.

treacle. Molasses.

trifolium. Used in eye diseases, clysters, fomentations.

triphora. Genus of American orchids.

triturated. Ground to powder.

trocar de minis. A trocar was a sharp rod fitting into a tube. Both were inserted into a body cavity, then the rod was withdrawn, allowing fluid to escape through the tube. *De minis*, of smaller size.

troche. Round pill.

troches alhandl. Troches of *Cucumis colocynthis*, a watermelon-like vine. Cathartic.

turbith. Turpeth, *Ipomoea*, morning glory. Cathartic.

tutty. Tutia, zinc oxide.

ung. diapomphol. *Unguentum diapompholigos*, ointment of oil of nightshade, white wax, washed beeswax, burnt lead, pompholix, and frankincense.

ungt. Arippe. Probably *unguentum Agrippae*, q.v.

ungt. martiatum. Soldier's ointment. Contained bay leaves, rue, marjoram, mint, sage, wormwood, basil, oil, wax, and wine.

ungt. *Unguentum*, ointment.

unguentum aegyptiacum. *Ceratum cetacei*, ointment of whale oil, white wax, and olive oil.

unguentum Agrippe. Briony roots, cucumbers, squill, orris root, fern root, dwarf elder, arum, oil, wax.

unguentum album. See *unguentum aegyptiacum*.

unguentum apostolorum. Had thirteen ingredients.

unguentum Arrogan. *Unguentum Arregon*, made with rosemary, marjoram, thyme, rue, bear's grease, etc.

unguentum basilicon. Wax, pitch, suet, turpentine, olibanum, myrrh.

unguentum de artanita. *Arthanita*, cyclamen. Purgative ointment.

unguentum de bolo. Bolo may have referred to *bole Armenian*, a clayey earth, or to *Boletus*, a fungus. Both were used as styptics.

unguentum dialthea. Composed of *Althaea*, linseeds, fenugreek seeds, wax, rosin, and turpentine.

unguentum Egyptiae. See *unguentum aegyptiacum*.

unguentum e nicotiana. Ointment of tobacco, made from tobacco leaves and juice, wine, rosin, birthwort, and wax. "It would take a whole Summer's day to write the particular vertues of this ointment" (p. 224).

unguentum fridg. Galeni. A cooling ointment of white wax, oil of roses, and rose vinegar.

unguentum populeum. Anodyne ointment containing buds of *Populeus*, the poplar, poppy leaves, belladonna, hyoscyamus, and black nightshade.

unguentum rosatum. Ointment of roses. Fresh hog's grease and roses were heated together and strained. To the juice was added oil of almonds and a little opium.

unguis oculi. Pterygion, a fleshy growth of the conjunctiva.

ungul. *Ungula*, claw, hoof.

vademecum. Go with me. A notebook or personal manual.

valet. It is strong.

Venice treacle. Molasses.

verbane. See *Verbena officinalis*.

Verbena officinalis. Vervain, used for headaches.

verdigrease. Verdigris, copper acetate.

ver. oris. Perhaps for *Veratrum*, false hellebore, a powerful emetic and purgative. Also used in anti-itching ointment. Or for *Viride aeris*, verdigris. See *verdigrease*.

vesicant. Producing blisters.

vesicatory. See *vesicant*.

vid. *Vide*, see.

Vinca pervinca. Periwinkle. Astringent.

vinegar of squills. *Acetum scillae*, made of vinegar and *Scilla*, squill. Diuretic, expectorant, emetic.

vini malvitici. *Vinum malviticum*, malmsey wine.

viola. Violet.

virga aurea. Golden rod, *Solidago*. Diuretic, stimulant.

Virginia snakeweed. *Aristolochia serpentaria*. Tonic, stimulant.

vir. oris. See *ver. oris*.

vitriolate. Sulphate.

vitriolum album. Zinc sulphate.

vulnerary. Remedy which facilitates wound healing.

wallwort. *Urtica*, common nettle. Juice was used in anodyne ointment.

wasted. Reduced in volume or amount.

watching. Wakefulness.

water caltrops. *Trapa natans*, water chestnut. Nut was considered soothing, demulcent. Also used in poultices for tumors.

water lilly. *Nymphaea*. Leaves are mucilaginous.

waters of angelica. See *aqua angelica*.

water of quick limes. Probably the liquid resulting when water is poured on quicklime. Applied to ulcers.

wen. A sebaceous cyst. Formerly also a wart or similar growth.

wether. Castrated ram.

white copperas. Zinc sulphate.

wormwood. *Artemisia*. Tonic, anthelmintic.

wormwood wine. Absinthe, brandy flavored with wormwood.

yard. Penis.

yarrow. *Achillea*. Used in dyspepsia, flatulence, hemorrhage, etc.

zeadeary. Probably *Zedoria, Kaempferia rotunda*, a Ceylonese plant. Roots are aromatic.

Bibliography

Ackerknecht, Erwin H. 1973. *Therapeutics from the Primitives to the Twentieth Century* . . . . New York: Hafner.

Adams, Francis, 1939. *The Genuine Works of Hippocrates* . . . . Baltimore: Williams & Wilkins.

Addy, William. [1690?]. *Stenographia or the Art of Short-Writing* . . . . London: Printed for the author.

Arnold, Dr. [n.d.] "*Brevis physicae appendix.*" MS.

Austin, Robert B. [1977]. *Early American Medical Imprints 1668–1820.* Arlington, Mass.: The Printer's Devil.

Barrough, Philip. 1601. *The Method of Phisick* . . . . London: Richard Field.

Beall, Ortho T., Jr., and Richard H. Shryock. 1954. *Cotton Mather: First Significant Figure in American Medicine.* Baltimore: Johns Hopkins Press.

Beinfield, Malcolm S. 1942. The Early New England Doctor: An Adaptation to a Provincial Environment. *Yale J. Biol. Med.* 15:99–132, 271–88.

Boorde, Andrew. 1547. *The Breviary of Helthe.* London: W. Middleton.

Bright, Timothy. 1588. *Characterie. An Arte of Shorte, Swifte, and Secrete Writing by Character.* London: I. Windet.

Brock, C. Helen. 1980. The Influence of Europe on Colonial Massachusetts Medicine. In *Medicine in Colonial Massachusetts, 1620–1820,* ed. P. Cash et al., pp. 101–16. Boston: Colonial Society of Massachusetts.

Cash, Philip, et al. eds. 1980. *Medicine in Colonial Massachusetts, 1620–1820.* Boston: Colonial Society of Massachusetts.

Chance, Burton. 1931. 'Nicholas Culpeper, Gent: Student in Physick and Astrologie'; 1616–1653–4. *Ann. Med. Hist.*, n.s. 3:394–403.

Cooke, James. 1648. *Melleficium chirurgiae* . . . . London: Samuel Cartwright.

———. 1655. *Supplementum chirurgiae* . . . . London: John Sherley.

Copeman, W. S. C. 1960. *Doctors and Disease in Tudor Times.* London: Dawson's.

Cowen, David L. 1956. The Boston Editions of Nicholas Culpeper. *J. Hist. Med. Allied Sci.* 11:156–65.

Culpeper, Nicholas. 1649. *A Physicall Directory* . . . . London: Peter Cole.

———. 1675. *Pharmacopoeia Londinensis* . . . . London: George Sawbridge.

———. 1708. *The English Physitian* . . . . London: P. Cole.

Debus, Allen G. 1965. *The English Paracelsians.* London: Oldbourne.

————, ed. 1974. *Medicine in Seventeenth-Century England*. Berkeley: University of California Press.

Dunglison, Robley. 1868. *A Dictionary of Medical Science* . . . . Philadelphia: H. C. Lea.

Eccles, Audrey. 1982. *Obstetrics and Gynaecology in Tudor and Stuart England*. Kent State, Ohio: Kent State University Press.

Eggleston, Edward. 1901. *The Transit of Civilization* . . . . New York: Appleton.

Erichsen-Brown, Charlotte. 1979. *Use of Plants for the Past 500 Years*. Aurora, Ontario: Breezy Creeks Press.

Estes, J. Worth. 1980. Therapeutic Practice in Colonial New England. In *Medicine in Colonial Massachusetts, 1620–1820*, ed. P. Cash et al., pp. 289–383. Boston: Colonial Society of Massachusetts.

Fernald, Merritt L., ed. 1950. *Gray's Manual of Botany*. New York: American Book Company.

Flück, Hans. 1976. *Medicinal Plants*. London: W. Foulsham.

French, John. 1651. *The Art of Distillation* . . . . London: R. Cotes.

Fuller, Thomas. 1710. *Pharmacopoeia Extemporanea* . . . . London: B. Walford.

————. 1723. *Pharmacopoeia Domestica* . . . . London: G. & J. Innys.

Gerarde, John. 1597. *The Herball or General Historie of Plantes*. London: E. Bollifant.

Gesner, Conrad. 1551–87. *Historia animalium*. Tiguri: apud C. Froschoverum.

Gifford, George E., Jr. 1980. Botanic Remedies in Colonial Massachusetts, 1620–1820. In *Medicine in Colonial Massachusetts, 1620–1820*, ed. P. Cash et al., pp. 263–88. Boston: Colonial Society of Massachusetts.

Gordon, Maurice B. 1949. *Aesculapius Comes to the Colonies* . . . . Ventnor, N.J.: Ventnor Publishers.

Guerra, Francisco. 1962. *American Medical Bibliography, 1639–1783*. New York: L. C. Harper.

Harrington, Thomas F. 1903. Dr. Samuel Fuller of the Mayflower (1620), the Pioneer Physician. *Bull. Johns Hopkins Hosp.* 14:263–70.

Harris, Ben C. 1972. *The Compleat Herbal* . . . . Barre, Mass.: Barre Publishers.

Holmes, Oliver W. 1911. *Medical Essays, 1842–1882*. Boston: Houghton Mifflin.

Jones, Gordon W., ed. 1972. *The Angel of Bethesda, by Cotton Mather*. Barre, Mass.: American Antiquarian Society and Barre Publishers.

Josselyn, John. 1672. *New Englands Rarities Discovered* . . . . London: G. Widdowes.

Kelly, Howard A. 1912. *A Cyclopedia of American Medical Biography* . . . . Philadelphia: Saunders.

Leighton, Ann. 1970. *Early American Gardens* . . . . Boston: Houghton Mifflin.

LeStrange, Richard. 1977. *A History of Herbal Plants*. London: Angus & Robertson.

Marks, Geoffrey, and Beatty, William K. 1973. *The Story of Medicine in America*. New York: Scribner's.

Mather, Cotton. 1689. *Memorable Providences, Relating to Witchcrafts and Possessions* . . . . Boston: R. P[ierce].

————. 1692. *Balsamum vulnerarium ex Scriptura* . . . . Boston: B. Green.

————. 1700. *The Great Physician* . . . . Boston: Timothy Green.

————. 1722. *The Angel of Bethesda*. New London: Timothy Green.

Moore, Norman. 1908. Fuller, Thomas. In *Dictionary of National Biography*, ed. S. Lee, vol. 7, pp. 760–61. New York: Macmillan.

Munk, William. 1878. *The Roll of the Royal College of Physicians of London* . . . . London: The College.

Murdock, Kenneth B. 1933. Cotton Mather. In *Dictionary of American Biography*, ed. D. Malone, vol. 12, pp. 386–89. New York: Scribner's.

Oliver, John. 1694. *A Present to Be Given to Teeming Women* . . . . Boston: B. Harris.

Packard, Francis R. 1931. *History of Medicine in the United States*. New York: Hoeber.

Poynter, F. N. L. 1962. Nicholas Culpeper and His Books. *J. Hist. Med. Allied Sci.* 17:152–67.

Read, John. 1966. *Prelude to Chemistry* . . . . Cambridge, Mass.: M. I. T. Press.

Rivière, Lazare. 1706. *Riverius reformatus* . . . . London: R. Wellington.

Rolls, Roger. 1982. Bark, Blisters, and the Bathe: Some Problems of Pain Relief in Former Times. *J. Roy. Soc. Med.* 75:812–19.

Royal College of Physicians. 1618. *Pharmacopoeia Londinensis*. London: E. Griffin.

Schroeder, Johann. 1649. *Pharmacopoeia medico-chymica* . . . . Ulmae: J. Gerlini.

Shryock, Richard H. 1960. *Medicine and Society in America, 1660–1860*. New York: New York University Press.

Steiner, Walter R. 1903. Governor John Winthrop, Jr., of Connecticut, as a Physician. *Bull. Johns Hopkins Hosp.* 14:294–302.

Sydenham, Thomas. 1848. *Works*. London: Sydenham Society.

Thacher, James. 1967. *American Medical Biography* . . . . New York: Milford House.

Thacher, Thomas. 1678. *A Brief Rule* . . . . Boston: J. Foster.

Thoms, Herbert. 1967. *Jared Eliot, Minister, Doctor, Scientist, and His Connecticut*. Hamden, Conn.: Shoe String Press.

Turner, William. 1551–68. *A New Herball.* London: S. Mierdman.

Viets, Henry R. 1930. *A Brief History of Medicine in Massachusetts.* Boston: Houghton Mifflin.

Vincent, Thomas. 1668. *God's Terrible Voice* . . . . Cambridge: M. Johnson.

Wigglesworth, William C. 1980. Surgery in Massachusetts, 1620–1800. In *Medicine in Colonial Massachusetts, 1620–1820,* ed. P. Cash et al., pp. 215–46. Boston: Colonial Society of Massachusetts.

Wirtzung, Christopher. 1617. *The General Practice of Physicke* . . . . Translated by Jacob Mosan. London: Thomas Adams.

Woodall, John. 1617. *The Surgion's Mate.* London: E. Griffin.

Woody, MacIver, to Janet Doe, 11 June 1953. In *Author Catalogue of the New York Academy of Medicine,* vol. 43, p. 287, Q 10153. Boston: G. K. Hall, 1969.

Index

The page numbers are those of this volume.